Public Health Evaluation and the Social Determinants of Health

Compelling evidence shows health disparities are the result of inequalities in income, education, limited access to medical care, substandard social environments, and poor economic conditions. This book introduces these social determinants of health (SDOH), discusses how they relate to public health programs, and explains how to design and evaluate interventions bearing them in mind.

Arguing that many public health programs fail to be as effective as they could be, because they ignore the underlying causes of health disparities, this important reference gives concrete examples of how evaluations focusing on the social determinants of health can alleviate health inequalities, as well as step-by-step guidance to undertaking them.

This resource blends current research, existing data, and participatory evaluation methods. It is designed for teachers, students, practitioners, and policymakers interested in public health programming and evaluation.

Allyson Kelley is an Evaluation Scientist with interests in building community capacity to address the cultural, social, and environmental factors that contribute to differences in health. Her interests are driven by what communities identify as most important. She leads evaluation efforts for several initiatives in Montana, Wyoming, South Dakota, and New Mexico. She has mentored more than 125 undergraduate and graduate students in the areas of evaluation and research methods. Dr. Kelley uses a community-based participatory approach and socioecological theories to guide her work.

Dr. Kelley is a trainer, speaker, author, and advocate of public health. In 2018 she published her first text, *Evaluation in Rural Communities*, published by Routledge. She currently serves as an Assistant Editor for the *International Journal of Doctoral Studies* and an Adjunct Assistant Professor at the University of North Carolina Greensboro in the School of Health and Human Sciences. She is a reviewer for several peer reviewed journals including the *American Journal of Public Health*, the *American Journal of Evaluation*, and the *American Indian Alaska Native Mental Health Journal*.

Dr. Kelley's work has resulted in numerous peer review publications, book chapters, and unpublished evaluation reports that highlight the importance of SDOH and public health evaluation approaches. Her efforts have resulted in new ways to build capacity, address determinants, and promote health equity in populations throughout the United States. She spends most of her time in New Mexico and Oregon and loves to hike, read, and rest.

Routledge Studies in Public Health

www.routledge.com/Routledge-Studies-in-Public-Health/book-series/RSPH

Available titles include:

Global Health Geographies
Edited by Clare Herrick and David Reubi

The Intersection of Food and Public Health
Current Policy Challenges and Solutions
Edited A. Bryce Hoflund, John C. Jones, Michelle Pautz

Conceptualising Public Health
Historical and Contemporary Struggles over Key Concepts
Edited by Johannes Kananen, Sophy Bergenheim, Merle Wessel

Global Health and Security
Critical Feminist Perspectives
Edited by Colleen O'Manique and Pieter Fourie

Women's Health and Complementary and Integrative Medicine
Edited by Jon Adams, Amie Steel, Alex Broom and Jane Frawley

Managing the Global Health Response to Epidemics
Social Science Perspectives
Edited by Mathilde Bourrier, Nathalie Brender and Claudine Burton-Jeangros

The Anthropology of Tobacco
Ethnographic Adventures in Non-Human Worlds
Edited by Mathilde Bourrier, Nathalie Brender and Claudine Burton-Jeangros

Public Health Evaluation and the Social Determinants of Health
Allyson Kelley

Public Health Evaluation and the Social Determinants of Health

Allyson Kelley

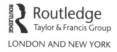
Routledge
Taylor & Francis Group

LONDON AND NEW YORK

First published 2020
by Routledge
2 Park Square, Milton Park, Abingdon, Oxon OX14 4RN

and by Routledge
52 Vanderbilt Avenue, New York, NY 10017

Routledge is an imprint of the Taylor & Francis Group, an informa business

British Library Cataloguing-in-Publication Data
A catalogue record for this book is available from the British Library

Library of Congress Cataloging-in-Publication Data
A catalog record has been requested for this book

ISBN: 978-0-367-41887-8 (hbk)
ISBN: 978-0-367-49866-5 (pbk)
ISBN: 978-1-003-04781-0 (ebk)

Typeset in Times New Roman
by Wearset Ltd, Boldon, Tyne and Wear

This book is dedicated to my mom. Thank you for teaching me that life's obstacles can be overcome by faith, grace, and believing in ourselves and others.

Contents

Figures

Tables

Preface

Stranded in the Denver airport for 24 hours due to ice, fog, and holiday travel, I watched people. Weather made all of us powerless over our ultimate goal of getting to our final destination. Fast forward 24 hours. The weather improved, most arrived at their destinations and went forward with holiday plans, the weather delay was a minor setback. But many, whose limited financial resources do not allow for unexpected costs, experience distress not felt by others.

This text is not about being stranded in an airport, but there are lessons that we can learn from this experience. Some believe that our health is determined by a lack of resources and money. Others feel health is driven by power, resources, and prestige. The social determinants of health combine socioeconomic determinants and structural determinants like policies and power to explore what determines health in people and populations throughout the world.

The goal of this book is to encourage evaluators, program staff, private organizations, government organizations, educators, students, and community members to integrate a social determinants of health (SDOH) focus into public health program evaluation. In doing this, we will transfer power to the individuals, communities, and populations that want health the most, but are the least empowered to achieve it.

Organization of text

I organized this book based on SDOH literature and evaluation methods. The first two chapters provide context and information about evaluation and the history of SDOH in the world. Chapter 3 describes planning SDOH evaluations and various approaches used. Chapter 4 describes how to collect and analyze SDOH data using examples from the US and around the world. Evaluation challenges and solutions are presented to prepare the reader for real-world SDOH evaluation. Chapter 5 describes several programs that utilize a SDOH focus and summarizes examples of private-sector funding to address SDOH. Health in All Policies is a cornerstone of this chapter and supports an evidence-based, equity-focused approach. Chapter 6 includes examples of SDOH evaluations from the literature and the author's experiences in the field. These examples demonstrate how programs impact structural inequalities and illustrates SDOH pathways that impact health. Chapter 7 is a case study that highlights how to conduct a SDOH evaluation and describes potential data sources and impacts. This book concludes in Chapter 8 with a summary of SDOH evaluation approaches, challenges, and solutions, and real-world application for evaluators wanting to build health equity in our world.

Pedagogical features

Each chapter begins with a quote or story that reinforces the chapter narratives. Chapters contain history, examples, and evidence on SDOH from the field. Each chapter ends with a summary and points to remember. Additional readings and resources provide more information on specific topics covered in the chapter. Chapter questions are designed to reinforce topics presented and methods used. Activities on the web are designed to engage students in learning about SDOH, data available, and real-world SDOH evaluation examples and programs. References are included at the end of each chapter. The appendix includes examples that readers can benefit from, an evaluation report outline, assessment tools, theory of change, logic model, health impact assessment, and health impact tracking matrix.

1 An overview of public health evaluation and the social determinants of health

Learning objectives

After reading this chapter, you should be able to:

- Define evaluation, program evaluation, and the types of evaluation used in public health
- Define the social determinants of health (SDOH) and provide examples
- Summarize the history of SDOH and key events leading up to advocacy for health as a fundamental human right
- List organizations involved in SDOH efforts
- Understand why SDOH focused evaluations are needed

In 1854, John Snow, a British physician, traced the source of a cholera outbreak in Soho, London, to a water pump handle. Snow had the water pump handle removed and cases of cholera immediately decreased (British Broadcasting Corporation, 2014). Some of you probably recognize his name and contributions as the beginning of modern epidemiology. Snow talked with residents of London and identified the source of the outbreak as a public water pump. Because Snow connected place and people, he was able to decrease mortality from the outbreak. Snow's early life was anything but privileged. He likely did not have economic stability, access to quality health care, acceptance by his community or peers, access to reliable transportation, or access to safe drinking water, clean air, or toxin free environments. Snow lived until the age of 45, and this was considerably longer than the average life expectancy for males born in 1813, estimated at 35 years (Office for National Statistics, 2015).

You might be wondering what John Snow's life has to do with public health program evaluation (PHE) and the social determinants of health … and the answer is everything. Public health seeks to improve the quality of life in individuals, families, and communities through the creation of social and physical environments that promote health for all people (Harris, 2016).

Evaluation as process is about finding value, through the systematic collection of information about activities, characteristics, and outcomes that allow us to make judgments about a program. Judgments help improve a program's effectiveness and inform decisions about how the program continues and develops (Centers for Disease Control and Prevention [CDC], 2011). Evaluation also helps determine value based on acceptable standards. An example of acceptable standards might be a target population health status and rates of morbidity and mortality within a community compared with state, national, or global average rates or norms. Evaluation occurs in a variety of contexts, but for the purposes of this text we will focus on PHE. In the United States, the Government Accountability Office defined **program evaluation** as a systematic study using research methods to assess how well a program works and why it works. Evaluation results assess effectiveness and identify how to improve programs or inform resource allocation and future efforts. PHE may be focused on a specific problem, initiative, or policy, or on an entire program.

Evaluation may be informal or formal. **Informal evaluation** might occur spontaneously when changes are needed to improve a program immediately—for example, changing program times, adding sessions, or revising how data is collected. **Formal evaluations** are systematic and well planned. Formal evaluations are characterized by planned activities, prescribed procedures and protocols, objective scores of measurement, controlled settings, narrowed scope, and strong inferences (McKenzie, Neiger, & Smeltzer, 2005).

Evaluation approaches are often identified by the terms process, outcome or impact, or formative and summative evaluations. Cost–benefit and cost-effectiveness evaluations are additional types of program evaluations frequently used in public health programming (Longest, 2014).

Process evaluations are used to determine if a program or part of a program is working as planned. Data collection for process evaluation may include information about services available, kinds of services provided, the extent to which these were delivered as planned, the social and demographic characteristics of individuals involved in programming, information about the community(ies) involved in a program, and the number and types of organizations involved in a given program. Results from process evaluations are used to identify needs, make changes, and redirect programming or service delivery. Process evaluations occur during program implementation. Sometimes process evaluation is called formative or implementation evaluation—for this text we will use the term process evaluation.

Outcome evaluations assess whether a program, policy, or initiative goal was met and if a program (or activity/component being evaluated) impacted a desired variable or outcome. Outcome evaluations often use a comparison group and compare results across a sample or population to determine the effect; and they occur after a program has been implemented or when there are outcomes available to compare. Sometimes outcome evaluation is called impact or summative evaluation. In this text we will use the term outcome evaluation.

Cost–benefit evaluation is used to determine the costs of operating a program in relation to the benefits of that program to an individual or society.

Cost-effectiveness evaluation is used to compare costs of operating a program to reach program goals and objectives.

Evaluation may be carried out internally by a program manager or staff member, or externally by an independent evaluator, expert, or funding agency. Evaluation standards may vary by program and context, but the Centers for Disease Control and Prevention (2017) developed 30 standards that guide program evaluation. Here are four categories used to organize standards: **Utility** ensures that an evaluation will serve the needs of the users or audience for which it is intended; **Feasibility** ensures that evaluations are realistic, prudent, diplomatic, and frugal; **Propriety** ensures that evaluations are legal, ethical, and consider those affected by evaluation results and involved in the program; and **Accuracy** ensures that evaluations communicate adequate information to help determine the worth or merit of a program (CDC, 2017).

The SDOH are focused on policies, programs, places, and people at the local, state, nation, or global level. PHE can help guide SDOH programming to document how efforts interact to create health or the absence of health (Krech, 2012). Combined, PHE and the SDOH have the potential to change the landscape of health in our lives and in our world. Throughout this text we will learn about the SDOH by exploring programs, policies, initiatives, and people. We will focus on how PHE can change the narrative about what determines health and how programs are addressing the underlying causes of health inequalities. Let's begin with exploring the history of SDOH.

Health as a universal right

The Universal Declaration of Human Rights (www.un.org/en/universal-declaration-human-rights/) affirms the equal and universal rights to health for all people, irrespective of economic class, gender, race, ethnicity, caste, sexual orientation, disability, age, or location. The right to health has been a topic of interest since the beginning of time. Without health, we die. With health, we live. But one of the challenges of public health is to find out why some people are healthy and live long lives, while others are not and do not. John Snow's efforts in the 1850s improved how people lived by ensuring residents of Soho, London, had safe drinking water, effective sewage disposal, food safety, housing, and safe work environments (Scriven & Garman, 2007). How do we know that Snow's work led to improved health? Using concepts and methods from PHE and efforts like Snow's we can provide evidence needed to advocate for policy changes that improve population health.

SDOH and history

There are some key events that led to a focus on SDOH as the primary driver of health equality and inequality—let's explore these now.

The constitution of the World Health Organization (WHO) was first drafted in 1946. This constitution was developed to address the social roots of health problems globally, and to address challenges related to medical care delivery. Their goal was that all people would attain the highest possible level of mental, physical, and social well-being.

Increasing costs of health care and "diseases of comfort" in the 1970s prompted new efforts to promote public health while addressing determinants of health. Public health in the United Kingdom (UK) and Canada changed radically with the release of the Lalonde Report (Lalonde, 1974). This was the first government document to recognize the importance of upstream policy agendas. Lalonde (1974) stated that improvements in health would come from improving the environment, moderating risk-taking behaviors, and increasing knowledge about human biology. A shortcoming of this report is that it resulted in an emphasis on lifestyle factors, on people taking responsibility for their own health, and a failure to address the socioeconomic and environmental factors that determine health.

The Alma Ata Declaration in 1978 proceeded from the Lalonde report. It was developed at the National Conference on Primary Health Care in Alma Ata, USSR (now called Almaty, Kazakhstan). This gathering of world health leaders, including WHO, was the first of its kind because it linked primary health care as a major factor in attaining the highest possible level of health for all people. This declaration also outlined steps to reduce health inequalities between countries and the role of governments in ensuring health as a fundamental human right.

The *Black Report*, published by the UK Department of Health and Social Security, documented inequalities in health and identified social factors— income, education, housing, diet, employment, and conditions of work—as the leading cause (Gray, 1982).

WHO's 1985 Health for All approach paved the way for health policy reform and a new focus on addressing population health through the socioeconomic determinants of health (WHO, 1986).

The 1986 International Conference on Health Promotion in Ottawa, Canada, followed the Alma Ata Declaration and resulted in the Ottawa Charter (WHO, 1986). The Ottawa Charter was designed to advocate for social justice and access to health, and to reduce health inequalities.

England attempted to follow health strategy reform with the Health of the Nation (HOTN) strategy published in 1992 (Department of Health, 1992). This strategy was lauded for being the first of its kind to promote health in a broad sense. But it was criticized because it failed to address the socioeconomic determinants of health and utilized a disease-based model of health, focusing on factors that contributed to diseases as opposed to the conditions that created them in the first place (Holland & Stewart, 1998).

President Clinton's 1998 health initiative targeted ethnic health disparities and called for health officials to address disparities. As a result of this initiative, Healthy People 2010 goals focused on research and policy interventions (Gehlert, Sohmer, Sacks, et al., 2008).

The Minority Health and Health Disparities Research and Education Act of 2000 prompted the creation of the Center for Minority Health and Health Disparities (US Department of Health and Human Services [USDHHS], 2000). This Center was, and is, charged with the development of the National Institutes of Health (NIH) Strategic Plan to address health disparities. Each institute at NIH has its own plan that addresses health disparities and the SDOH.

The Institute of Medicine's USA report (IOM, 2002) found that the US was failing in the area of population health and called for collective action. The IOM report defined health as a primary public good and emphasized human potential, relationships, and political participation. Without health, humans are unable to participate or contribute to society in a meaningful way.

Wilkinson and Marmot (2003) published the 10 solid facts about SDOH. This seminal paper documented the link between social and economic conditions and poor health. These and other SDOH will be explored throughout this text.

In 2008, the WHO Commission on SDOH called for local action on the SDOH with the aim of achieving health equity. The Commission challenged health care practice and traditional public health approaches by asking, "What good does it to do to treat people's illnesses and send them back to the same conditions that made them sick?" The report from WHO provided three recommendations for achieving health equity within one generation:

- Improve daily conditions
- Tackle the inequity distribution of power, money, and resources
- Measure and understand the problem and assess the impact of action (WHO, 2008)

Then in 2010, following the WHO Commission on SDOH, Lancet led an effort to develop a new vision for health professionals to address SDOH using institutional strategies and competency-based approaches (Frenk et al., 2010).

Following the WHO Commission and Lancet efforts, the Rio Political Declaration on SDOH was adopted by 120 member states (National Academies of Sciences, Engineering, and Medicine [NAS], 2016). This landmark event resulted in collective action to address SDOH throughout the world. The WHO Commission created nine knowledge networks to improve areas for SDOH action. These are as follows:

- Early childhood development and education
- Employment and working conditions
- Health care and health systems
- Urban settings
- Globalization
- Social Exclusion
- Women and gender equity
- Priority public health conditions
- Measurement and evidence (WHO, 2008)

In 2017 WHO, National Children's Fund, and the Rio Political Declaration on the SDOH called for evaluation of SDOH interventions that improve health equity. This relatively recent call is one of the primary reasons that this textbook was conceptualized and written.

The US Department of Health and Human Services (USDHHS) focuses on SDOH in its population health model and in 2019 the USDHHS Commission on SDOH called for increasing health care worker knowledge about SDOH. Using Healthy People 2020 (www.healthypeople.gov/2020/topics-objectives/topic/social-determinants-health/interventions-resources) as a guide, the SDOH are organized into five place-based domains: economic stability, education, health and health care, neighborhood and built environment, and social/community context. These will be defined later in this chapter.

What are the SDOH?

WHO defines SDOH as "the conditions in which people are born, grow, live, work, and age." (WHO, 2019). These conditions are most often determined based on an individual's or community's ability to access resources, money, and power. Conditions are responsible for the differences in health observed within and between countries throughout the world (WHO, 2019). Table 1.1 compares the SDOH noted in some of the US and global milestones described above.

How we talk about the SDOH matters. In the UK, these population differences are defined as **inequalities** among groups based on socioeconomic status and conditions (Marmot & Allen, 2014). In the US, the term **disparities** is often used and refers to the racial and ethnic differences in health care. **Health equity** is a term used to describe fairness and justice as they relate to the SDOH. In this text we will use all these terms and explore SDOH from multiple social pathways that guide population health across communities and countries.

Health policies and programs, health factors, and health outcomes are attributable to our physical, social, economic, health care, and health behaviors. Health follows a social gradient; as socioeconomic position increases, health improves (WHO, 2008). Healthy People 2020 organizes the SDOH based on five domains:

- Economic stability
- Education
- Health and health care
- Neighborhood and built environment
- Social and community context

Let's explore these SDOH pathways in the next sections.

Economic stability

Social and economic factors such as community safety, family and social support, income, employment, and education account for 40% of one's quality of life and length of life (Robert Wood Johnson Foundation [RWJF], 2014).

Income and wealth. Economic resources affect health, and income inequality has been associated with health. Factors such as educational attainment and

Table 1.1 Comparison of SDOH US and global

	United Kingdom Black Report	*WHO 1986 Ottawa Charter for Health Promotion*	*WHO 2003 10 Solid Facts*	*WHO 2016 Rio Political Declaration on SDOH*	*United States Healthy People 2020*
SDOH Domains and Focus Areas	Income, education, housing, diet, employment, and conditions of work (Gray, 1982)	Peace, shelter, education, food, income, stable ecosystem, sustainable resources, social justice, and equity (WHO, 1986: Ottawa Charter).	Social gradient, stress, early life, social exclusion, work, unemployment, social support, addiction, food, and transport (Wilkinson & Marmot, 2003).	Early childhood development and education, employment and working conditions, health care and health systems, urban settings, globalization, social exclusion, women and gender equity, priority public health conditions, measurement and evidence (WHO, 2019).	Economic stability, education, health and health care, neighborhood and built environment, and social/ community context (USDHHS, 2000).

quality, childhood socioeconomic status (SES), neighborhood characteristics, working conditions, and subjective social status are associated with income and wealth. Economic instability also affects health. In 2016, more than 40.6 million people lived in poverty, or 12.3% of the US population (US Census Bureau, 2017). Low SES is related to increased risk for the following diseases: cardiovascular disease, arthritis, diabetes, chronic respiratory disease, cervical cancer, and mental distress.

Occupation, employment status, and workplace safety. Physical and psychosocial, and social, aspects of where we work can influence our health. Previous research has found that the work environment affects an individual's risk for injuries and disorders, obesity, and obesity-related conditions. The physical environment that an individual works in can also affect health—consider ventilation and noise levels. Psychosocial aspects of working conditions can include high-demand and low-control work environments, perceived imbalance of efforts and rewards, and the social aspects of work and support received and offered to and from co-workers. In addition, employment income and benefits impact health-related decisions for individuals and families.

Education

Education affects health knowledge and health behaviors. Education also creates employment opportunities, which are then linked to economic opportunities that affect health. Education also influences the social and psychological factors that are associated with health. Moreover, educational attainment affects an individual's sense of control, social standing, and social support (Braveman, Egerter, & Williams, 2011). Previous studies have demonstrated a graded relationship between the mother's educational attainment, her life expectancy, and infant mortality of her children—as educational attainment increases, life expectancy increases and infant mortality decreases (Braveman et al., 2011).

Health and health care

Access to care and quality of health care one receives accounts for 20% of one's quality of life and length of life (RWJF, 2014). Lack of health insurance coverage is a primary barrier to health care access, and this affects health (Office of Disease Prevention and Health Promotion, 2019). Vulnerable populations are at high risk for inadequate health insurance coverage, and low income and minorities account for more than 50% of the uninsured population in the US. However, health insurance coverage is not enough to improve population health or social well-being (de Andrade, Pellegrini Filho, Solar, et al., 2015).

Neighborhood and built environment

Physical environment, including air and water quality, housing, and transit, accounts for 10% of one's quality of life and length of life (RWJF, 2014).

Neighborhood-level effects impact health and are associated with elevated rates of intentional injury, poor birth outcomes, cardiovascular disease, HIV, gonorrhea, tuberculosis, depression, physical inactivity, and all-cause mortality (Krieger & Higgins, 2002). Other research has documented that where we live determines mortality, low birth weight, depression, cancer, and cardiovascular disease (Ross, 2000). Our physical environment also predicts how we engage with the world around us, form relationships, and interact socially—all of these determine our health (Ross, 2000).

Access to housing and utility services. Previous research has demonstrated that where we live impacts our health. Housing is linked to the social gradient, in that the lower an individual is on the social gradient, the more substandard their housing will be. Dunn and colleagues explored housing dimensions by socioeconomic factors and found vulnerabilities among subpopulations (Dunn, Hayes, Hulchanski, et al., 2006). Poor housing is associated with numerous health conditions including respiratory infections, asthma, lead poisoning, injuries, and poor mental health (Krieger & Higgins, 2015). Substandard housing may create physical hazards, exposure hazards, inadequate ventilation, or stress due to the location. Other dimensions of housing include overcrowding and homeless populations.

Availability of transportation. When people have limited access to reliable transportation it impacts their health. Hispanics, Latinos, African Americans, and Asian Americans are more likely to report just one vehicle per household compared to Whites. Lower income minorities are more likely to use public transit and carpools than Whites. This results in more time spent trying to get from one location to another.

Access to safe drinking water, clean air, and toxin free environments. Marmot and colleagues found that the where people live is impacted by the socioeconomic gradient (Marmot, Allen, Bell, et al., 2012). At lower levels, the built environment is often substandard, unhealthy, and people are more likely to be exposed to tobacco smoke, biological and chemical contamination, hazardous waste sites and dumps, air pollution, flooding, fires, poor sanitation, noise pollution, and road traffic (WHO, 2010).

Recreation and leisure opportunities. Physical inactivity is associated with increased risk of all-cause mortality. Gonzalo-Almorox and Urbanos-Garrido (2016) conducted a cross-sectional study of the Spanish National Health Survey and found a significant socioeconomic gradient associated with recreation and leisure time. This same study found that lower parental educational attainment and incomes were associated with physical inactivity in Spanish youth. Recreation and leisure have several health benefits, but if one's health or socioeconomic status does not allow participation in such opportunities because of lack of education, working long hours, or unsafe neighborhood environments, then health inequalities will be observed.

Food insecurity and inaccessibility of nutritious food choices. Limited access to food (food insecurity) is a risk factor for several diseases including obesity, chronic kidney disease, diabetes, and hypertension (Banerjee, Crews,

Wesson, et al., 2017). Consumption of ready-to-eat products or ultra-processed foods is associated with neighborhood-level socioeconomic status. When people do not have the resources to purchase, prepare, and store healthy foods, they are more likely to consume unhealthy foods. Leite and colleagues conducted a study on the association of neighborhood food availability in Santos, Brazil, and found that when children lived in lower SES neighborhoods, they were more likely to consume unhealthy processed foods (Leite, de Carvalho Cremm, de Abreu, et al., 2018).

Social and community context

Health behaviors such as tobacco use, diet and exercise, alcohol and drug use, and sexual activity account for 30% of one's quality of life and length of life (RWJF, 2014).

Early childhood experiences and development. Where children are born determines their health, in terms of their exposure to sustained poverty, abuse and neglect, parental alcohol or drug abuse, homelessness, and family violence. The first eight years of life are considered the most sensitive to the SDOH (Moore, McDonald, Carlon, et al., 2015).

Social support and community inclusivity. Social or relational support benefits mental health. Social support improves mental health, can strengthen family resilience, and enhances community connections (Shim, Ye, Baltrus, et al., 2012). Lack of social support can lead to feelings of stress, depression, and disconnectedness, impacting health.

Crime rates and exposure to violent behavior. Crime follows a social gradient, and low-income neighborhoods are more likely to report higher crime and victimization rates than higher-income neighborhoods (Kang, 2016). When people feel uncertain about their physical security and fear violence, they are more likely to stay in their homes (Office of Disease Prevention and Health Promotion, 2019). This increases their exposure to toxins found in the indoor environment and decreases physical activity, which contributes to obesity and poor mental health.

Gender inequality. Girls and women across the world experience physical and mental health impacts because they are viewed as unequal to their male counterparts. Some have defined the root causes of gender inequality as the most influential SDOH of our time. Gender, in many cases, determines our voice in the health sector, in society, and where one is on the social gradient. In the US, for example, women earn 77 cents for every $1.00 that men earn (DeNavas-Walt, Proctor, & Smith, 2009). Despite major strides in the last 100 years to promote gender equality in the workplace and schools, there is still a lack of equality. Gender systems, structural processes, and the structural determinants of health create conditions that affect people's health.

Racial segregation. Racism is a determinant of health and is associated with poorer mental and physical health, even after controlling for age, sex, birthplace, and education (Paradies, Ben, Denson, et al., 2015). Racial residential segregation is an example of institutional racism that contributes to social disadvantage in neighborhoods with limited resources (Bharmal, Derose, Felician, et al., 2015). Research indicates that racism impacts health through stress pathways (Szanton, Rifkind, Mohanty, et al., 2012). Harris and colleagues explored racism and health from the New Zealand Health Survey of 12,500 people (Harris, Tobías, Jeffreys, et al., 2006). They found that racial discrimination was significantly associated with poor or fair self-rated health, lower physical functioning, lower mental health, smoking, and cardiovascular disease. There was a graded relationship between the number of types of discrimination and each health measure.

More than just determinants

Researchers and agencies agree that health is determined by multiple factors happening at the same time, or throughout a lifespan. Consider the landmark study by McGinnis and Foege (1993). They identified the causes and numbers of death in the year 1990 and found that half of the deaths could be attributed to nongenetic factors such as tobacco, diet/activity patterns, alcohol, and firearms. Their work prompted public health professionals to think differently about health and the interplay of individual behaviors, social environment or characteristics, environmental conditions, and health services and health care (McGinnis & Foege, 1993). Similarly, Galea and colleagues conducted a meta-analysis of almost 50 studies in the United States—they found that more than one-third of deaths each year are attributed to income, education, social supports, and racial segregation (Galea, Tracy, Hoggatt, et al., 2011). Therefore, when thinking about the SDOH, think broadly and explore interrelated determinants of health.

Organizations that lead SDOH efforts

Remember John Snow from the beginning of this chapter? He may not have known that his work would be linked to the SDOH or public health. Public health in our world now is led by WHO, the Centers for Disease Control and Prevention, communities, and, in the US, the DHHS. Then come organizations like the American Public Health Association, World Bank, United Nations Children's Fund, United States Agency for International Development, and nongovernmental organizations like Doctors Without Borders, CARE International, and Population Services International.

The **World Health Organization (WHO)** was created by the United Nations system in 1948. The initial goals of WHO were to address malaria, tuberculosis, venereal disease, and other communicable diseases while improving women's and children's health. Other priorities related to nutrition and sanitation. Geneva, Switzerland, is the headquarters for WHO and there are 194 countries that are members of WHO across six regions in the world. WHO is well known for its work to address river blindness and eradicate smallpox. However, WHO efforts to address HIV/AIDS have been criticized for being too slow, and not doing enough (WHO, 2019).

The **Department of Health and Human Services in the United States**, originally the Department of Health, Education and Welfare (HEW), was created in 1953 by President Eisenhower. Then, in 1979, the Department of Education was removed and the DHHS was created. DHHS' goal is to protect the health of all Americans and provide services to populations that are unable to help themselves. DHHS oversees the Centers for Medicare and Medicaid Services, the Food and Drug Administration, the NIH, and the Centers for Disease Control and Prevention.

The **Centers for Disease Control and Prevention (CDC)** was founded by Dr. Joseph Mountin in Atlanta, Georgia. On July 1, 1946 the Communicable Disease Center opened for business. Its primary goal was to prevent malaria. Today CDC funding exceeds 7.3 billion dollars, with 35% of its funding geared toward protecting Americans from infectious disease. Other CDC functions include monitoring health and laboratories, safety in the workplace, protection from natural and bioterrorism threats, ensuring global disease protection, and preventing causes of disease, disability, and death (CDC, 2019). CDC works with state, local, county, and community partners to implement various public health functions.

Organizations, individuals, and communities throughout the world are working to address health as a fundamental human right. This work will not happen overnight, and it will not be the work of just one organization—but the collective.

The case for SDOH and answering the call

Sir Michael Marmot calls for action—it is matter of social justice. SDOH is one of WHO's six priority areas (Marmot & Allen, 2014). Education on SDOH within the workforce, professionals like you and me, is needed to address critical workforce shortages and the lack of distribution of skills in the current health workforce (NAS, 2016). Since the 2011 World Conference on the SDOH, and the adoption of the Rio Political Declaration on the SDOH by 120 member states, progress has been made. There are several governments, organizations, and ministries responding to the SDOH call. Foundations like the Robert Wood Johnson Foundation and the Kellogg Foundation fund SDOH initiatives throughout the US and world, initiatives that are changing the landscape of public health.

The WHO Commission on SDOH, the Rio Political Declaration on SDOH, and European reviews and assessments on SDOH (health inequities) call for policy action in these areas:

- Policies that directly influence socioeconomic living conditions that affect health and health inequities
- Policies for improving healthcare provision and coverage
- Actions to improve governance arrangements within and between countries to support and enable the effective implementation of these policies (Saunders, Barr, McHale, et al., 2017)

Policies are in progress. In the US, these are evident in the Health Impact in 5 Years initiative, Health in All Policies, urban design, and transportation policies and practices. Evaluation of such SDOH programs is emerging. One example is the evaluation of early childhood programs that invest in educational and development resources for disadvantaged families, at the Heckman Equation— evidence shows a 13% return on investment for birth-to-five programs (Heckman Equation, 2019). We will learn even more about policies, PHE, and SDOH later in this text. Stay tuned.

Evaluation: Why focus on SDOH?

> Evaluation is a systematic approach for determining the value of something.
> (American Evaluation Association, 2014)

There is a place for SDOH in evaluation because it guides the value seeking process. Professionals who evaluate programs are empowered to guide public health policy, research, social justice, and interventions that build health equality and equity. This text marks a paradigm shift in how public health approaches evaluation from a SDOH lens.

I believe we have wasted precious time. Time in public health, in com-munities, and with people that could be better used to address the underlying causes of inequalities. Some have referred to this as the causes of the causes. To date, most evaluations that include SDOH have been cross-sectional in nature, and they have failed to link a determinant to a health outcome. Why? Because causality has always been a challenge, but especially when it comes to multiple causes, multiple communities, multiple unknowns, power, structures, and politics. Public health evaluators are challenged with navigating this landscape. We will learn more about these challenges and potential solutions later in this text.

In sum, we cannot change what we do not acknowledge. If we, as public health professionals, ignore SDOH in evaluation, then we will fail to address the causes of the causes. The time is now, for public health to set aside evaluations that solely document progress, input, activities, outputs, outcomes, and impacts without getting to the underlying causes of health inequalities and injustice in our world.

We are at a pivotal point in time politically, economically, and structurally. Some have referred to this as a tipping point. What are you willing to do? I say we start focusing on the SDOH, the conditions, geographies, policies, structures, and populations that influence health.

Summary

We began this book and this chapter by reading about John Snow's work in public health. He saved thousands of lives by removing a water pump handle that was exposing people to cholera. At the time, many people doubted his theory of disease and thought cholera was airborne and not waterborne. Snow's germ theory of disease was eventually accepted in the 1860s. Snow died in 1858 from a stroke. He never witnessed the full impact of his efforts on the field of public health.

Understanding the historical context of health, SDOH, and how different countries and organizations promote health is a first step in public health evaluation that utilizes a SDOH approach. In this chapter we learned about how organizations define public health, strategies, centers, and initiatives designed to address SDOH, but are they working? The SDOH defined in this chapter are interrelated with causality pointing in multiple directions toward health or the absence of health. What history tells us is that it is now time for a shift in how we promote health and address the widening health gap in our world.

Points to remember

1   The history of SDOH can tell us what not do to, and point to areas of what to do to address health inequalities and promote justice.
2   Organizations throughout the world are addressing the SDOH through policy change, workforce development, education, technical assistance, research, and advocacy efforts.
3   SDOH is about social justice.
4   More than one-third of all deaths are attributable to the SDOH.
5   Public health professionals play an important role in answering the call to action and closing the health gap throughout the world.
6   Evaluation of public health programs that address the SDOH is one way that evidence, policy, and change can happen.

Additional reading and resources

American Evaluation Association Online Handbooks and Texts
www.eval.org/p/cm/ld/fid=79

Centers for Disease Control and Prevention
www.cdc.gov

Centers for Disease Control and Prevention Evaluation Framework Resources
www.cdc.gov/eval/framework/index.htm

World Health Organization
www.who.int/

Chapter questions

1   Compare and contrast the types of evaluations listed at the beginning of this chapter.
2   List the four categories that guide evaluation standards. How might these standards be useful in PHE that focuses on the SDOH?

3   List functions of WHO and their role in addressing the SDOH in countries throughout the world.

4   Summarize the history of SDOH and the agencies involved in addressing SDOH presented in this chapter.

5   Reflect on the different types of SDOH summarized in this chapter. Which SDOH has the most potential to improve public health? Which has the least?

6   What three recommendations resulted from the 2008 WHO report for achieving health equity in one generation? How might these be achieved? What are the challenges for addressing these?

Activities on the web

1   Identify three separate initiatives that support health as a human right. For example, health care as a human right (see: https://dignityandrights.org/our-work/). Describe the initiatives you selected and discuss which SDOH they are most closely associated with.

2   Conduct a web search of health organizations that are addressing the SDOH throughout the world. List five organizations not mentioned in this chapter. Summarize their work and their SDOH focus.

References

American Evaluation Association. (2014). *What is evaluation?* Retrieved from: www.eval.org/p/bl/et/blogid=2&blogaid=4.

Banerjee, T., Crews, D. C., Wesson, D. E., Dharmarajan, S., Saran, R., Burrows, N. R., ... & McCulloch, C. (2017). Food insecurity, CKD, and subsequent ESRD in US adults. *American Journal of Kidney Diseases*, 70(1), 38–47.

Bharmal, N., Derose, K., Felician, M., & Weden, M. (2015). *Understanding the upstream social determinants of health.* RAND Health. Retrieved from: www.resourcebasket.org/wp-content/uploads/2019/01/upstream.pdf.

Braveman, P., Egerter, S., & Williams, D. R. (2011). The social determinants of health: Coming of age. *Annual Review of Public Health*, 32, 381–398.

British Broadcasting Corporation (BBC). (2014). History. John Snow. Retrieved from: www.bbc.co.uk/history/historic_figures/snow_john.shtml.

Centers for Disease Control and Prevention. (2011). *Introduction to program evaluation for public health programs: A self-study guide.* Retrieved from: www.cdc.gov/eval/guide/index.htm.

Centers for Disease Control and Prevention. (2017). CDC evaluation framework index. Retrieved from: www.cdc.gov/eval/framework/index.htm.

Centers for Disease Control and Prevention. (2019). CDC funding and history. Retrieved from: www.cdc.gov/about/report/index.html.

de Andrade, L. O. M., Pellegrini Filho, A., Solar, O., Rígoli, F., de Salazar, L. M., Serrate, P. C. F., ... & Atun, R. (2015). Social determinants of health, universal health coverage, and sustainable development: Case studies from Latin American countries. *The Lancet*, 385(9975), 1343–1351.

DeNavas-Walt, C., Proctor, B. D., & Smith, J. C. (2009). *Income, poverty, and health insurance coverage in the United States: 2008.* Current population reports: Consumer income. Washington, DC: US Census Bureau. Retrieved from: www.census.gov/prod/2009pubs/p60-236.

Department of Health. (1992) The health of the nation: A strategy for health in England. Her Majesty's Stationery Office. Available from: https://navigator.health.org.uk/content/health-nation-%E2%80%93-strategy-health-england-white-paper-was-published.

Dunn, J. R., Hayes, M. V., Hulchanski, J. D., Hwang, S. W., & Potvin, L. (2006). Housing as a socio-economic determinant of health: Findings of a national needs, gaps and opportunities assessment. *Canadian Journal of Public Health/Revue Canadienne de Santé Publique, 97*(Suppl. 3), S11–S15.

Frenk, J., Chen, L., Bhutta, Z. A., Cohen, J., Crisp, N., Evans, T., … & Zurayk, H. (2010). Health professionals for a new century: Transforming education to strengthen health systems in an interdependent world. *The Lancet, 376*(9756), 1923–1958.

Galea, S., Tracy, M., Hoggatt, K., DiMaggio, C., & Karpati, A. (2011). Estimated deaths attributable to social factors in the United States. *American Journal of Public Health, 101*(8), 1456–1465. doi:10.2105/AJPH.2010.300086.

Gehlert, S., Sohmer, D., Sacks, T., Mininger, C., McClintock, M., & Olopade, O. (2008). Targeting health disparities: A model linking upstream determinants to downstream interventions. *Health Affairs, 27*(2), 339–349.

Gonzalo-Almorox, E., & Urbanos-Garrido, R. M. (2016). Decomposing socio-economic inequalities in leisure-time physical inactivity: The case of Spanish children. *International Journal for Equity in Health, 15*(1), 106.

Gray, A. M. (1982). Inequalities in health. The Black Report: A summary and comment. *International Journal of Health Services, 12*(3), 349–380. doi:10.2190/XXMM-JMQU-2A7Y-HX1E.

Harris, M. J. (2016). *Evaluating public and community health programs.* Retrieved from https://ebookcentral.proquest.com.

Harris, R. B., Tobías, M., Jeffreys, M., Waldegrave, K., Karlsen, S., & Nazroo, J. (2006). Racism and health: The relationship between experience of racial discrimination and health in New Zealand. *Social Science & Medicine, 63*(6), 1428–1441.

Heckman Equation. (2019). *The economics of human potential.* Retrieved from: https://heckmanequation.org/.

Holland, W. W., & Stewart, S. (1998). Public health: Where should we be in 10 years? *Journal of Epidemiology and Community Health, 52*(5), 278.

Institute of Medicine. (2002). Understanding population health and its determinants. In *The future of the public's health in the 21st century* (pp. 46–95). US Committee on Assuring the Health of the Public in the 21st Century. Washington, DC: The National Academies Press. Retrieved from: www.ncbi.nlm.nih.gov/books/NBK221225/.

Kang, S. (2016). Inequality and crime revisited: Effects of local inequality and economic segregation on crime. *Journal of Population Economics, 29*(2), 593–626.

Krech, R. (2012). Working on the social determinants of health is central to public health. *Journal of Public Health Policy, 33*(2), 279–284.

Krieger, J., & Higgins, D. L. (2002). Housing and health: Time again for public health action. *American Journal of Public Health, 92*(5), 758–768.

Lalonde, M. (1974). *A new perspective on the health of Canadians.* Ottawa, Canada: Information Canada.

Leite, F. H. M., de Carvalho Cremm, E., de Abreu, D. S. C., de Oliveira, M. A., Budd, N., & Martins, P. A. (2018). Association of neighbourhood food availability with the consumption of processed and ultra-processed food products by children in a city of Brazil: A multilevel analysis. *Public Health Nutrition, 21*(1), 189–200.

Longest, B. (2014). *Health program management: From development through evaluation.* Retrieved from https://ebookcentral.proquest.com.

Marmot, M., & Allen, J. (2014). Social determinants of health equity. *American Journal of Public Health, 104*(Suppl. 4), S517–S519.

Marmot, A., Allen, J., Bell, R., Bloomer, E., & Golblatt, P. (2012). WHO European review of social determinants of health and the health divide. *The Lancet, 380*(9846), 1011–1029.

McGinnis, J. M., & Foege, W. H. (1993). Actual causes of death in the United States. *JAMA, 270*(18), 2207–2212.

McKenzie, J., Neiger, B., & Smeltzer, J. (2005). *Planning, implementing, and evaluating health promotion programs: A primer* (4th ed.). San Francisco, CA: Pearson/Benjamin Cummings.

Moore, T., McDonald, M., Carlon, L., & O'Rourke, K. (2015). Early childhood development and the social determinants of health inequities. *Health Promotion International, 30*(Suppl. 2), ii102–ii115.

National Academies of Sciences, Engineering, and Medicine. (2016) *A framework for educating health professionals to address the social determinants of health.* Washington, DC: The National Academies Press. doi:10.17225/21923.

Office for National Statistics. (2015). *How has life expectancy changed over time?* Retrieved from: www.ons.gov.uk/peoplepopulationandcommunity/birthsdeathsandmarriages/ lifeexpectancies/articles/howhaslifeexpectancychangedovertime/2015-09-09.

Office of Disease Prevention and Health Promotion. (2019). SDOH interventions and resources: Access to health services. Retrieved from: www.healthypeople.gov/2020/topics-objectives/topic/social-determinants-health/interventions-resources/access-to-health.

Paradies, Y., Ben, J., Denson, N., Elias, A., Priest, N., Pieterse, A., … & Gee, G. (2015). Racism as a determinant of health: A systematic review and meta-analysis. *PLoS ONE, 10*(9), e0138511.

Robert Wood Johnson Foundation. (2014). County health rankings model. Retrieved from: www.countyhealthrankings.org/county-health-rankings-model.

Ross, C. E. (2000). Neighborhood disadvantage and adult depression. *Journal of Health and Social Behavior, 41*(2), 177–187.

Saunders, M., Barr, B., McHale, P., & Hamelmann, C. (2017). Key policies for addressing the social determinants of health and health inequities. Health Evidence Network (HEN) synthesis report 52. Copenhagen, Denmark: WHO Regional Office for Europe.

Scriven, A., & Garman, S. (2007). *Public health: Social context and action.* Retrieved from https://ebookcentral.proquest.com.

Shim, R. S., Ye, J., Baltrus, P., Fry-Johnson, Y., Daniels, E., & Rust, G. (2012). Racial/ ethnic disparities, social support, and depression: Examining a social determinant of mental health. *Ethnicity & Disease, 22*(1), 15.

Szanton, S. L., Rifkind, J. M., Mohanty, J. G., Miller, E. R., Thorpe, R. J., Nagababu, E., … & Evans, M. K. (2012). Racial discrimination is associated with a measure of red blood cell oxidative stress: A potential pathway for racial health disparities. *International Journal of Behavioral Medicine, 19*(4), 489–495.

US Census Bureau. (2017). *Income and poverty in the United States.* Report P60-259. Available from: www.census.gov/library/publications/2017/demo/p60-259.html.

US Department of Health and Human Services. (2000). *Healthy People 2010: Understanding and improving health.* Washington, DC: US Government Printing Office.

Wilkinson, R. G., & Marmot, M. (Eds.). (2003). *Social determinants of health: The solid facts*. World Health Organization. Retrieved from: https://books.google.com/books?hl=en&lr=&id=QDFzqNZZHLMC&oi=fnd&pg=PA5&dq=marmot+and+wilkinson+2003&ots=xVuJfBURju&sig=vgWIEX1gQapfhyZaHYcydGGFkCM#v=onepage&q=marmot%20and%20wilkinson%202003&f=false.

World Health Organization. (1946). *Constitution of the World Health Organization*. Geneva, Switzerland: WHO.

World Health Organization. (1986). *Ottawa Charter for Health Promotion*. Geneva, Switzerland: WHO.

World Health Organization. (2008). *Closing the gap in a generation: Health equity through action on the social determinants of health, final report*. Geneva, Switzerland: WHO Commission on Social Determinants of Health.

World Health Organization. (2010). *Environment and health risks: A review of the influence and effects of social inequalities*. Copenhagen, Denmark: WHO Regional Office for Europe.

World Health Organization (2011). *Rio Political Declaration on Social Determinants of Health*. World Conference on Social Determinants of Health. Rio De Janeiro Brazil, October 2011. Available from: www.who.int/sdhconference/declaration/Rio_political_declaration.pdf

World Health Organization. (2019). *Social determinants of health: Countries*. Retrieved from: www.who.int/.

2   A condition of place, people, communities, and justice

Learning objectives

After reading this chapter, you should be able to:

* Define upstream, midstream, and downstream determinants of health
* List the six essential elements of well-being
* Summarize racial categories and unique populations as they relate to SDOH
* Describe the relationship between place and health

Upstream, midstream, and downstream people, places, and conditions

This is what we know. Current approaches to improve health inequities among people, places, and conditions are not as effective as they need to be. We can stand by rivers of flowing waters and not know what is upstream.

> There I am standing by the shore of a swiftly flowing river and I hear the cry of a drowning man. So I jump into the river, put my arms around him, pull him to shore and apply artificial respiration. Just when he begins to breathe, there is another cry for help. So I jump into the river, reach him, pull him to shore, apply artificial respiration, and then just as he begins to breathe, another cry for help. So back in the river again, reaching, pulling, applying, breathing then another yell. Again and again, without end, goes the sequence. You know, I am so busy jumping in, pulling them to shore, applying artificial respiration, that I have no time to see who the hell is upstream pushing them all in.
>
> (Zola, cited in McKinlay, 1979, p. 9)

When we utilize the SDOH, this is an upstream approach—the goal is to determine why people are in the river in the first place. Unfortunately, some of public health has focused on a medical model that focuses on the treatment of diseases through medical care and traditional health outcomes rather than focusing on the social and environmental factors that impact health (McKinlay, 1979).

Addressing upstream causes is a population-level approach to improving public health for all. The upstream approach focuses on prevention or intervention strategies that could potentially save an entire population from falling into a river. The downstream approach, on the other hand, involves pulling one person at a time from the river, and individually treating them. Often upstream interventions involve policy, increased access, or economic incentives (Brownson, Seiler, & Eyler, 2010).

Overview and narrative of concepts

Sir Michael Marmot (2005) writes and speaks about population-level determinants using the example of social status gradient that determines health outcomes in populations. Marmot and other researchers have demonstrated that social status defined by the gradient impacts an individual's risk of heart disease onset. They found that the social status gradient was independent of an individual's biological risk for developing heart disease (Marmot, 2005).

The NIH-sponsored Centers for Population Health and Health (CPHH) called attention to addressing health disparities as a primary public health goal through a multilevel research agenda that addresses determinants of health disparities. Warnecke and colleagues wrote about NIH's initiative to create a new paradigm that would address health disparities through multilevel, transdisciplinary research (Warnecke, Oh, Breen, et al., 2008). From this initiative, eight CPHH Disparities were established (2003–2008). Centers called for a population health approach to health disparities and created a model for analyzing population health and health disparities (see Warnecke et al., 2008, p. 1611). Within this model they identified three primary types of determinants that are often used to understand the distribution of health outcomes in a population. **Distal determinants** are population social conditions, policies that affect these conditions, policy makers or policy-making organizations that are responsible for addressing social conditions. **Intermediate determinants** include social and physical environments and social relationships. Examples include neighborhood or community poverty, residential segregation, income, education, social interactions (Diez-Roux, Nieto, Muntaner, et al., 2017). The physical environment often determines access to health care resources, transportation, air and water quality, and healthy food, as well as crime, violence, and the extent to which disparities in health outcomes are observed. **Proximal determinants** include individual demographics, risk behaviors, biological responses, and biological genetic pathways. The interaction of these determinants affects one's capacity to respond to social and environmental conditions that impact health. Consider the example of biological markers that document elevated cholesterol after prolonged exposure to stress—these proximal factors are likely the result of heredity, environmental stress, and behavior (Elliott, 2000).

Warnecke and colleagues (2008) make clear that population-level determinants (distal determinants) are different from individual-level health outcomes (determined by proximal factors)—often these population-level determinants are expressed as rates, percentages, distributions, and patterns of segregation. In contrast, individual-level determinants relate to risk factors like one's educational attainment, income, or genetic makeup.

Arah and colleagues conducted a pooled cross-sectional time series analysis for member countries of the Organisation for Economic Cooperation and Development (OECD) from 1970 to 1999 (Arah, Westert, Delnoij, et al., 2005). They found that all-cause mortality and potential years of life lost (PYLL) decreased 37% across the selected countries. PYLL is used to estimate the number of years that a person would have lived if they had not died prematurely. Proximal determinants of protein and fruit/vegetable consumption increased while those of alcohol, tobacco, and fat intake decreased. Immunization levels and collective health expenditure also increased. Distal determinants of healthcare coverage levels improved by about 2 to 4 percentage points after excluding the United States from the estimates. Intermediate determinants measured by elderly populations, national wealth, density of practicing physicians, and doctor visits during the 1970–1999 period increased. This study was the first to document the impact of tobacco, alcohol, fat, fruit/vegetable, air pollution, collective health expenditure, healthcare coverage, and immunizations on mortality and premature death (Arah et al., 2005).

Upstream midstream downstream. What matters? How do we address the causes of the causes? Public health interventions occur at multiple levels, not just the individual level. Let's take a closer look (and see Figure 2.1, which illustrates the upstream downstream concept).

- Upstream interventions target systems change and often involve policy approaches that affect large populations through regulation, increased access, or economic incentives. Consider the 1964 campaign by the Surgeon General that advised people about the harmful effects of tobacco

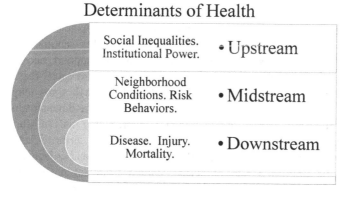

Figure 2.1 Upstream downstream SDOH.

use. This campaign is related to decreases in smoking that have been observed for the last 50 years (National Research Council, 2004). Another example of an upstream intervention is increasing tobacco taxes to control tobacco-related diseases (Thomson, Hillier-Brown, Todd, et al., 2018).

- Midstream interventions often occur within organizations or communities. Midstream interventions are designed to change health behaviors by changing environmental conditions that support them (National Research Council, 2004). One example is a work-based wellness program that encourages employees to engage in physical activity (Song & Baicker, 2019).
- Downstream interventions involve individual-level behavioral approaches—and these are the most common level of intervention in the management or prevention of disease. disease. For example, programs that encourage people with diabetes to look after their health involve lifestyle changes such as exercising more and eating healthy foods, as well as medical changes like monitoring blood sugar levels. These lifestyle changes occur at the individual level (National Research Council, 2004).

Upstream

Upstream approaches are often viewed as more powerful for addressing SDOH than downstream measures; let's look at why.

Upstream conditions. These conditions give rise to policies that support equity and equality for all. Such policies aim to ensure that every individual and family has access to affordable housing, safe neighborhoods, fair standards of living, and healthy environments, and aim to eliminate racism. Upstream conditions include social inequities of class, race and ethnicity, immigration status, gender, and sexual orientation which can be linked to institutional inequities. Interventions that target upstream conditions target these institutional inequities, which are enmeshed with the macro factors that make up sociostructural influences on health and health systems, government policies, and the social, physical, economic, and environmental factors that determine health.

Consider Latino families living in the United States. They experience upstream challenges and conditions of poverty. This often means they may experience low income, high debts to assets ratios, and negative financial events. These factors make it difficult to access quality childcare, quality schools and education, safe neighborhoods, stable housing, social and legal support, access to healthy food, access to reliable transportation, and quality health care—these are upstream challenges that determine health. In fact, because Latinos may experience these upstream factors, they are likely to experience the downstream effects of the conditions of poverty. Latinos in the US report higher rates of heart disease, stroke, cancer, diabetes, respiratory conditions, obesity, arthritis, and pedestrian fatalities, all linked to conditions of poverty. Chaufan and colleagues at the University of California San Francisco studied upstream antecedent factors contributing to downstream health disparities in Latino immigrants associated with type 2 diabetes (Chaufan, Davis, & Constantino, 2011). In this study, upstream factors were food environment and poverty and the downstream factor was type 2 diabetes (T2DM). Their rationale for exploring antecedent factors was that the prevention and management of T2DM are based on access to healthy food environments. But many Latino immigrants receiving services at the non-profit organization they partnered with did not have access to healthy foods and 100% of Latinos in the study relied on some form of food assistance. They concluded that the right to healthy and adequate food is a fundamental human right because it supports the right to health, and they called for interventions that reduce T2DM from a social justice perspective.

Public policies have large effects on health behaviors, while individual and community-level interventions may not (National Research Council, 2004). Because of this, policy makers and public health professionals are calling for more focus on upstream factors to reduce health inequalities in our world. But, what does this look like? Due to the complexity of upstream factors, involving more than just one condition or social structure, intervention strategies grounded in SDOH have to address multiple upstream SDOH. Causal pathways are long and complex, involving multiple intervening factors, and this makes upstream causes difficult to evaluate and study in the field of public health. Yet upstream public health measures are needed to improve population health and promote health equity (Dover & Belon, 2019). But what about midstream and downstream …? Read on.

Midstream

Midstream conditions. The stream moves people from conditions that do not promote health or well-being to better stream conditions, conditions that support them and the conditions that they live in. Midstream conditions are supported by community-level actions. These conditions are good paying jobs, quality education, physical activity, access to health care, access to transportation, and access to environments that support healthy development and growth for all.

Let's consider the midstream condition of quality education. We know that education is associated with longer life expectancy, improved health and quality of life, healthy behaviors like exercise, not smoking, and getting regular health check-ups (Lahelma, Martikainen, Laaksonsen, et al., 2004). National initiatives like Healthy People 2020 aim to improve education quality and increase the proportion of students who graduate with a regular diploma in four years after starting ninth grade to 87% by 2020. Using common core data from the National Center for Educational Statistics, in 2010–2011, the adjusted cohort graduation rate (ACGR) was 79% for all students attending public schools. This rate increased to 85% during the 2016–2017 school year. However, differences in educational achievement remain across race and ethnicities. For example, Asian/Pacific Islanders have the highest ACGR of 91%, followed by White non-Hispanic or Latino students at 89%, Hispanic or Latino at 80%, Black or African American non-Hispanic or Latino at 78%, and American Indian Alaska Native at 72% (National Center for Education Statistics, 2019). Regional variations in ACGRs were also observed, where just 76% of White students in New Mexico graduated with a high school diploma compared with 95% of White students in New Jersey. What can we learn about the stream conditions in these states and schools that promote graduation rates or reduce them?

Downstream

Downstream conditions. Target communities or individuals. It is easy to focus on downstream conditions and this is what most health-related programs and interventions do. In public health, prevention may focus on primary, secondary, or tertiary approaches. Primary prevention is disease occurrence, secondary prevention is disease progression, and tertiary prevention is lessening the long-term effects and/or chances that the disease will reoccur. Medical research and health care delivery are all downstream public health approaches as well. The challenge with downstream public health approaches is that they focus on health outcomes rather than determinants of health outcomes, and therefore completely miss what is happening upstream (Carey & Crammond, 2015). Consider social isolation as a determinant of health. Research tells us that Black women are more likely to die from breast cancer than White women. They will develop cancer younger than White women (Carey, Perou, Livasy, et al., 2006). Why? Researchers believe that upstream factors create increased risk for certain types of cancers and that by knowing what these factors are ahead of time, public health interventions can close the mortality gap. When social interactions increase, hormone profiles linked to triple negative cancers (like breast cancer) decrease.

Conditions

What we know is that the stream conditions are interrelated and connected. Water that comes from upstream eventually travels down to the middle of the stream, and then further downstream. There are different ways that public health professionals can work in the stream. Consider the social and economic conditions combined with other structural factors that impact population health outcomes. Social gradients and health behaviors go hand-in-hand. A study of risky sexual behaviors in a rural North Carolina community found that lack of neighborhood resources (adequate recreational options, lack of safe environments/housing) led to an increase in risky sexual behaviors (Akers, Muhammad, & Corbie-Smith, 2011).

Social epidemiology

Recall from Chapter 1 our introduction to John Snow, the father of modern epidemiology. Well, social epidemiology stems from his early work but focuses on sociostructural factors that impact health. Examples of sociostructural factors from previous authors include social class, gender, race and ethnicity, dissemination, social network, social capital, income distribution, and social policy. One of the primary questions that guides the work of social epidemiologists is exploring what effect social factors have on individual and population health (Honjo, 2004). While this is not an epidemiology textbook, evaluators often borrow from other disciplines in their evaluation of public health programs, and therefore it is important to understand some key concepts in social epidemiology. The bio-psychosocial paradigm supports the assumption that health is determined by multiple factors at different time points. Population strategies are used in social epidemiology to explore the risk factors associated with the absence of health in a population rather than an individual. Statistical approaches can help explore the effects of the sociostructural factors mentioned previously on health. Rather than just looking at one sociostructural factor and one health outcome, multilevel modeling allows us to explore all variables at one time. Lastly, social epidemiology requires a theory to build a hypothesis about what is happening and why. This theory is then used to select variables of interest and develop conceptual frameworks about relationships between variables and health outcomes. Social epidemiology is critical for SDOH evaluations because we know that what determines health, or the absence of health, is the convergence of multiple streams, environments, risks, and protective factors.

Justice

Health is about justice and justice promotes well-being. The concept of injustice plagues the history of the United States, with groups being treated unjustly based on their race, ethnicity, gender, class, or other factors that make them "different" than the dominant culture and power. Consider the history of the United States: slavery, forced relocation and genocide of American Indian and Alaska Native peoples, limited rights of women, segregation laws, mass deportation of Hispanic immigrants, internment of Japanese Americans, exclusion policies to Chinese people, criminalization of homosexual behaviors, and the list goes on (Gee & Ford, 2011). In the early 1900s women who were White, and people of color, were not allowed to work in certain occupations and could not vote or run for political office. During this time, if you were disabled, you were often either discriminated against, institutionalized, or socially excluded. We have come a long way in the United States to create a just world, but one of the most glaring injustices that remains is the lack of health equity and equality across population groups.

Powers and Faden (2006) defined six essential dimensions of well-being: health, personal security, reasoning, respect, attachment, and self-determination. Social justice requires that society provides its members with the social conditions necessary to achieve these six dimensions of well-being. Public health is emerging as a key challenger of injustice in the world. Earlier in this chapter we learned that health is a fundamental human right. When people do not have access to streams that support this right, then the stream conditions must change, for they are unjust. The Network for Public Health Law (www.networkforphl. org/) advocates for health justice through public health and advancing health equity. Focus areas related to health justice include food insecurity as a health justice issue—when people do not have access to foods, or healthy foods, it is difficult to find health in the stream. Access to health care is also a health justice issue. Although the Affordable Care Act and other policy work has increased access and coverage, 28.5 million people in the US still do not have access to health care (Berchick, Hood, & Barnett, 2018). Homelessness is another health justice issue. The list of injustices related to health continues to grow with the widening gap between resource rich and resource poor individuals and countries. The gap widens by race and unique populations.

Race

In the United States, there are five racial categories: White, Black or African American, American Indian or Alaska Native, Asian, and Native Hawai'ian or other Pacific Islander. Hispanic and Latino are observed as ethnicities, not races (Office of Management and Budget, 2018). Health outcomes are determined by racial and ethnic group status at the national, state, and county level. Du Bois' early research on race and health in 1899 reported that poor health for Blacks was an indicator of racial inequality in the United States. DuBois and Eaton (1899) were the first authors to report racial differences as a reflection of the differences in social structure and conditions that favored Whites but not Blacks. Their findings have been repeated throughout time, where widespread differences in educational attainment are linked with poverty based on racial, ethnic, and geographic status. Blacks and Latinos, both socially disadvantaged groups, consistently experience poorer health outcomes than Whites. Researchers have found that racial disparities in health are related less to the biological factors of race, and more to the social factors, policies, and structures (Williams & Sternthal, 2010). A driver of racial disparities in health is racism that occurs at the individual, community, or structural level. Gee and Ford (2011) describe levels of structural racism using the iceberg metaphor, where individually mediated acts are something like a cross burning. The part of the iceberg that cannot be seen below the water represents structural racism—it is unseen, more dangerous, and difficult to target. Thus, structural racism may be at the macrolevel, within social forces, institutions, ideologies, policies, and processes that have converged to generate inequities among racial and ethnic groups. SDOH focused evaluations must consider structural racism and the implications it has for overall health outcomes, access to quality care, discrimination, and poverty.

Unique populations

The report *Communities in Action: Pathways to Health Equity* describes the state of health disparities in the United States and underlying causes of health inequities, including populations that are disproportionately impacted by health inequities (NAS, 2017). These populations include Native American, American

Indians or Alaska Natives, gender groups, Lesbian, Gay, Bisexual, and Transgender persons, veterans, and persons with disabilities.

Native Americans, American Indians, or Alaska Natives. There are 5.2 million American Indians or Alaska Natives living in the United States. There are 573 federal Indian Nations (also called tribes, nations, bands, pueblos, communities, and native villages). Within each Indian Nation there is rich diversity in language, history, customs, and traditions that have been passed down from generation to generation. Nations are sovereign and have a unique political status with the US government, the Indian Nation in which the state is located, and international rights (National Congress of American Indians, 2019). Treaties signed more than 100 years ago guaranteed access to federal health care services, and the Indian Health Service was developed based on these treaties, yet health care access and quality continues to lag behind what it needs to be. Native people report poorer health outcomes, higher mortality rates, and higher infant mortality rates than their White counterparts (Blue Bird Jernigan, Peercy, Branam, et al., 2015).

Gender groups. Differences in life expectancy among men and women are decreasing but remain an important area for SDOH focused intervention and evaluation. In 2016 a woman's life expectancy in the US was 81.0 years and a man's was just 76.1 years (National Center for Health Statistics, 2018). One of the key factors driving mortality increases in women is intimate partner violence—women are more likely than men to be injured in an assault (Tjaden & Thoennes, 2000). Over time, a woman's exposure to violence increases risk of arthritis, asthma, heart disease, gynecological problems, and risk factors for HIV or sexually transmitted diseases (STDs). Men of color may experience disproportionate amounts of community violence. Men also commit suicide more frequently than women for all age groups and racial or ethnic classifications—with rates four times greater than women (CDC, 2019). Recent research suggests that White women are more likely to die from opioid overdose deaths than men or other racial groups (CDC, 2019).

Lesbian, Gay, Bisexual, and Transgender persons. LGBT persons are considered sexual minorities because of their non-heterosexual sexual orientation (i.e., Lesbian, Gay, or Bisexual) or their gender identity such as Transgender. Sexual orientation and gender identity minorities are often referred to as LGBT as an umbrella term. This term encompasses other forms of sexual and gender expression that exist within this population, which are greater than the acronym suggests. Some of the challenges that LGBT populations experience relate to the "invisibility" of LGBT individuals and communities, and the forms of stigma and social and legal discrimination they encounter. Brown and Herman (2015) discuss the unique disparities of LGBT persons. Among Gay men, HIV and AIDS remain major threats to health. Bisexual persons are disproportionately impacted by intimate partner violence (Brown & Herman, 2015). Transgender persons experience disparities which are driven primarily by the SDOH. For example, Transgender women have difficulty finding employment and poverty can lead to sex work, which places them at risk for incarceration, violence, substance abuse, and HIV as well as other sexually transmitted infections.

Persons with disabilities. Physical, cognitive, or mental health–related impairments may affect health outcomes. There are 48.9 million people in the US, or 19.4% of the non-institutionalized civilian population, who have a disability; of these, 24.1 million have a severe disability. Mobility issues make up the largest percentage of people with functional disabilities, accounting for 13.7% of disabilities, followed by cognition disabilities, which make up 10.8% of all disability types (CDC, 2018). Evidence suggests that people with disabilities are likely to have poorer health outcomes, but data to document health disparities among people with disabilities has been difficult to identify because of the lack of consensus on what constitutes a disability (Oreskovich & Zimmerman, 2012).

Let's consider the discrimination against deaf people in the United States. Ann was born in 1944 in Salem Oregon. At the age of 6 she lost her hearing, and she believes her hearing loss could have been caused by having a high fever for several days. She never confirmed this with doctors because in the 1950s children like Ann living in poverty did not have access to medical care. Her family did not have the means to take her to a doctor because of her prolonged fever. Eventually Ann recovered from her illness and went back to school, where she was in the first grade. She never recovered her hearing loss, but she was too afraid to tell anyone that she could not hear. Relying on lip reading only, Ann navigated her way through elementary, middle, and part of high school. It was during high school that she finally had her hearing checked, as one of her teachers knew that she was not able to hear, despite Ann telling them she was fine. During this decade, there was a prevailing attitude that "deaf people were dumb" and Ann just wanted to be like all of her peers, without a disability. Ann was able to get medical help after hearing tests showed that she was legally deaf. Luckily, during the 1960s hearing aid technology was evolving from transistor hearing aids to digital hearing aids. Ann's family saved up enough money to buy one hearing aid, and from this her life changed dramatically. Ann learned sign language, navigated her silent environment by lip reading, and worked through college with the dream of becoming a teacher. She graduated with honors in 1973, but these honors were not enough at the time. Ann was considered unqualified to be a teacher because of her disability. Although disappointed, Ann went on to get her master's degree in teaching, thinking that this would supersede her disability status, and that she would finally be able to teach. Unfortunately, the degree did not matter, for systems in place in the Department of Education prohibited people with disabilities from becoming teachers in the State of Oregon. Fast forward 40 years. Although the 1990 Americans With Disabilities Act (ADA) prohibited discrimination based on disability status, millions of deaf people are still being discriminated against, turned down for work, because they have a disability. This means that organizations, societies, and systems believe that they are not enough. The 1990 ADA is simply not enough to address structural factors that reduce opportunity and disempower individuals with disabilities.

Veterans. Consisting of veterans of the armed forces, this population is predominantly male, with more education and financial means than the US general male population. As a population, the veterans experience different values, customs, and communication practices that are unique to a veteran culture. Veterans also experience mental disorders, substance use disorders, post-traumatic stress, and traumatic brain injuries at higher rates than the US population. Young veterans between the ages of 18 and 44 are at highest risk for suicide. Homelessness, chronic pain, depression, amputations, access to rehabilitation care, hazardous exposures, and access to quality health care are unique factors that this population experiences. The Veterans Health Administration (VHA) serves US veterans of the armed forces but has been plagued by health care crises for decades, with topics like patient safety, long wait times, cleanliness, leadership, lack of funding, lack of providers, and limited support for female veterans (Wax-Thibodeaux, 2018).

Consider all of the people that live by the stream, their gender, ethnicity, race, religion, disability, veteran status, sexual orientation, and geographic locations. How people engage with the world around them and with others determines health. When people are not connected socially with others, their ability to cope with social and/or environmental stressors decreases, and this dysregulates the physiological process that affects health outcomes downstream (Gehlert, Mininger, Sohmer, et al., 2008).

Places

We live in a big world, with multiple streams, multiple people, places, conditions, histories, structures. Previous work tells us that each of these places has a unique set of conditions that determines health. Although we do not know the precise mix, we know that health is determined by the convergence of stream conditions. Evidence demonstrating that where we live relates to how healthy we are and how long we live is not new. In the 1970s, researchers published studies that demonstrated associations between residential areas and all-cause mortality (Neser, Tyroler, & Cassel, 1971). The association between place and health as they relate to mortality, low birthweight, depression, cancer, and cardiovascular disease have been documented (Yen & Kaplan, 1999).

As I am writing this chapter I stand at a desk in the mountains of New Mexico. My world is very different from someone who is standing at a desk in London, New York City, or Swaziland. The place where we stand has a profound impact on our paradigm, how we view ourselves and the world around us, what determines health or takes away from health. The place where we stand also impacts our beliefs, goals, values, resources, and life course.

If we are to evaluate SDOH programs we must consider the places where we stand and how these places influence health. Twenty years ago, it was common for Indians in Bangladesh to go to a local stream to collect water for drinking, wash their clothes, provide water for livestock, or swim. But today, these streams are polluted with toxic trace metals, coliforms, and organic and inorganic pollutants. Use of streams for drinking, bathing, and washing clothes is not recommended by public health officials. Death due to waterborne diseases in Bangladesh is common and water pollution has a major impact on public health. Researchers indicate that identifying the point and non-point sources of pollution is what needs to happen to restore water quality. In the case of India, point sources are agricultural pollution and industrial or and chemical waste (Hasan, Shahriar, & Jim, 2019). Although technology to treat point sources is improving, it is costly, and requires policy change to ensure that all waste is treated before leaving the source. We can learn from the streams in India, to see that it is not enough to simply know pollution exists and public health is compromised. Actions are needed to address the risk and vulnerabilities of children, the elderly, and any individuals living in areas with limited resources or limited power to change the stream. Where we stand on the stream has everything to do with our ability and power to change the stream. Let's look at where rural Americans live on the stream.

Rural. Rural America experiences greater inequities in health than the rest of the nation. Individuals and families living throughout rural America report fewer resources, poorer health outcomes, and less education. Results from the Economic Research Services show a growing gap between metropolitan and non-metropolitan poverty rates from 1959 to 2016. Racial and ethnic group differences demonstrate that Black, American Indian/Alaska Native, and Hispanic populations in non-metro areas are more likely to experience poverty than their counterparts living in metro areas in the United States (Economic Research Service, 2018). Figure 2.2 illustrates this.

Rural counties have consistently had the highest premature death rates in the United States. They also experience higher rates of preventable conditions (such as obesity, diabetes, cancer, and injury), and higher rates of related high-risk health behaviors (such as smoking, physical inactivity, poor diet, and limited use of seatbelts) (Downey, 2013). Premature death due to poverty, isolation, discrimination, limited access to quality health care, lack of safe environments, community norms, and poor mental health are potential areas for SDOH focused evaluation.

Urban. Individuals living in urban places also experience health disparities. The food environment is one of the unique conditions of the urban locale, for

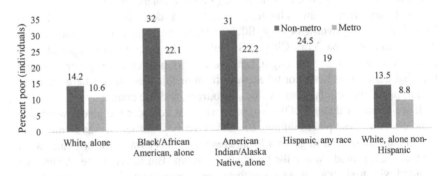

Figure 2.2 US poverty rates by race/ethnicity metro and non-metro residence 2017.

Source: Economic Research Service (2018).

food insecurity is most common among individuals that live in urban cities such as Chicago, Houston, Los Angeles, New York, and Phoenix (Gunderson & Ziliak, 2015). Violence is also higher in urban locations; a report from the Prevention Institute (nd) shows that two-thirds of all homicides with a firearm occur in urban areas and cities. Exposure to violence over time creates chronic stress, and chronic stress has been associated with anxiety, depression, and a multitude of other health challenges. Asthma is also more common in urban areas and this is partially due to air pollution, exposure to indoor and outdoor smoke, and pest allergens (Kozyrskyj, Kendall, Jacoby, et al., 2010).

Developing countries. Increasingly, public health professionals are focusing on developing countries to reduce the global health gap. The United Nations (UN) World Economic Situation and Prospects (WESP) provides classification status for all countries in the world. Classifications are based on three categories (developed economies, economies in transition, and developing countries) (UN, 2014). There are 49 developing countries in the world, most located in Africa, East Asia, South Asia, Western Asia, and Latin America and the Caribbean (UN, 2014). Children living in developing countries who come from poor families have higher risk of death than those from rich families. Current efforts in developing countries focus on maternal and child health, immunizations, and increasing health care access. Researchers have found that the largest intervention points are addressing economic inequalities that contribute to gaps in health outcomes (Amouzou, Kozuki, & Gwatkin, 2014).

Clearly upstream, midstream, and downstream approaches help us conceptualize how health equity might be achieved in populations throughout the world. However, conceptualizing such approaches is not enough. To fully understand the multiple factors that determine health inequities, we must explore these streams, changes to the stream, and health over time. Researchers at the National Academies of Sciences and several other leading research organizations (2017) reviewed what is known about SDOH and health inequities. They concluded that five steps are needed to promote upstream SDOH efforts.

- First, expand current health disparity indicators and indices to include unique groups listed in this chapter (recall racial and ethnic groups, gender groups, LGBT individuals, people with disabilities, and military veterans).
- Second, consider the best methods to document stable estimates of disparities. With smaller, unique populations, oversampling of certain populations may yield better outcomes for documenting the extent of health inequities in a given population.
- Third, create broad definitions of health that include health equity, SDOH, and justice.
- Fourth, conduct studies that explore how one structural factor can influence multiple health outcomes.
- Fifth, increase funding opportunities for examining structural inequities such as structural racism and health disparities.

Summary

In this chapter we have learned about the upstream, midstream, and downstream approaches to addressing SDOH. Understanding such approaches is a first step in planning SDOH focused evaluations that build health equity and equality across populations. This chapter explored the importance of place and health, along with unique populations that should be considered in SDOH focused evaluations beyond racial or ethnic classifications. One similar theme throughout multiple streams, places, and people is the relationship between poverty and health. Poverty cannot be viewed as the problem, but rather it must be viewed as a result of something much bigger. When individuals are not afforded the same opportunities, to attend quality schools, access quality health care, and receive fair and equal treatment as citizens of their countries (US or otherwise), this has a negative impact on health. Research from around the globe demonstrates that the gap between the rich and poor continues to grow, and that within this gap health inequities in populations that experience poverty continue to grow as well. Addressing the structural causes of persistent poverty, limited education, and poor living conditions is one way that SDOH focused evaluations can change the world. The changes will not happen overnight, but if we change the focus to see what is happening upstream, or, as in the story we started this chapter with, *who is pushing people into the river*, then we can change the stream conditions and what is possible to achieve through collective public health efforts that promote justice for all.

Points to remember

1   There are multiple approaches to SDOH focused evaluations. We conceptualized these in this chapter as upstream, midstream, and downstream. Where we stand on the stream, the quality of the water running through the stream, and what we do depends largely on how empowered we are or, in some cases, disempowered.

2   Unique populations exist in our world that deserve special attention as we pave the way for SDOH focused evaluations. Understanding how to incorporate these groups and their unique status in SDOH focused evaluation is a first step in building equality and empowerment for all.

3   Place plays an important role in how we live and our health outcomes. SDOH focused evaluations must recognize the role of place, the power structures, institutions, and policies that build or take away from the health of people.

Additional reading and resources

United Nations World Mortality 2017 Data Booklet
www.un.org/en/development/desa/population/publications/pdf/mortality/World-Mortality-2017-Data-Booklet.pdf

World Health Organization Mortality Database
www.who.int/healthinfo/mortality_data/en/
Centers for Disease Control Lesbian, Gay, Bisexual, and Transgender Health
www.cdc.gov/lgbthealth/
Rural Health Information Hub SDOH Resources
www.ruralhealthinfo.org/topics/social-determinants-of-health

Chapter questions

1 Compare and contrast upstream, midstream, and downstream conditions that impact health.
2 List unique population groups in the United States. Describe health disparities that they may experience based on their unique population status. Summarize how unique population status could be integrated into a SDOH focused evaluation approach.
3 Review place as it relates to health using rural, urban, and developing country status. Summarize health disparities and inequalities that individuals may experience living in these areas.
4 Write about where you stand, in relation to your own health. How does the place where you live, work, and socialize impact your health? Your paradigm? Your access to healthy activities and foods? Sense of community?

Activities on the web

1 Watch the video, *Unnatural Causes* (https://unnaturalcauses.org/about_the_ series.php). Select from one of the episodes from the list below and discuss how evaluations could potentially address inequalities and underlying causes of disease and health differences.
In Sickness and Wealth
When the Bough Breaks
Becoming American
Bad Sugar
Place Matters
Collateral Damage
Not Just a Pay Check
2 Visit the Institute for Health Metrics and Evaluation (IHME) Global Burden of Disease website (www.healthdata.org/gbd/data) and review data visualizations, country profiles, and publications. Discuss how these items of data demonstrate world health through demographic data. How might this data be helpful in developing a SDOH focused evaluation? What are some of the challenges?
3 Explore the UN Country Classification list (www.un.org/en/development/ desa/policy/wesp/wesp_current/2014wesp_country_classification.pdf). Describe the UN's classification methodology. Summarize differences in countries that export and import fuel, and in per capita gross national income;

identify heavily indebted poor countries. How might fuel, gross national income, and debt contribute to the health disparities in these countries?

References

Akers, A. Y., Muhammad, M. R., & Corbie-Smith, G. (2011). "When you got nothing to do, you do somebody": A community's perceptions of neighborhood effects on adolescent sexual behaviors. *Social Science & Medicine, 72*(1), 91–99.

Amouzou, A., Kozuki, N., & Gwatkin, D. R. (2014). Where is the gap? The contribution of disparities within developing countries to global inequalities in under-five mortality. *BMC Public Health, 14*, 216. doi:10.1186/1471-2458-14-216.

Arah, O., Westert, G., Delnoij, D., & Klazinga, N. (2005). Health system outcomes and determinants amenable to public health in industrialized countries: A pooled, cross-sectional time series analysis. *BMC Public Health, 5*, 81. doi:10.1186/1471-2458-5-81.

Berchick, E., Hood, E., & Barnett, J. (2018). Health insurance coverage in the United States 2017. United States Census Bureau. Retrieved from: www.census.gov/content/dam/Census/library/publications/2018/demo/p60-264.pdf.

Blue Bird Jernigan, V., Peercy, M., Branam, D., Saunkeah, B., Wharton, D., Winkleby, M., ... & Buchwald, D. (2015). Beyond health equity: Achieving wellness within American Indian and Alaska Native communities. *American Journal of Public Health, 105*(Suppl. 3), S376–S379. doi:10.2105/AJPH.2014.302447.

Brown, T., & Herman, J. (2015). Intimate partner violence and sexual abuse among LGBT people. Los Angeles, CA: The Williams Institute. Retrieved from: https://williamsinstitute.law.ucla.edu/wp-content/uploads/Intimate-Partner-Violence-and-Sexual-Abuse-among-LGBT-People.pdf.

Brownson, R. C., Seiler, R., & Eyler, A. A. (2010). Measuring the impact of public health policy. *Preventing Chronic Disease, 7*(4), A77.

Carey, G., & Crammond, B. (2015). Systems change for the social determinants of health. *BMC Public Health, 15*(1), 662. doi:10.1186/s12889-015-1979-8.

Carey, L. A., Perou, C. M., Livasy, C. A., Dressler, L. G., Cowan, D., Conway, K., ... & Deming, S. L. (2006). Race, breast cancer subtypes, and survival in the Carolina Breast Cancer Study. *JAMA, 295*(21), 2492–2502.

Centers for Disease Control and Prevention. (2018). Disability and health data system (DHDS) [updated 2018, May 24]. Retrieved from: http://dhds.cdc.gov.

Centers for Disease Control and Prevention. (2019). Web-based Injury Statistics Query and Reporting System (WISQARS). Atlanta, GA: National Centre for Injury Prevention and Control. Available online: www.cdc.gov/injury/wisqars/index.html.

Chaufan, C., Davis, M., & Constantino, S. (2011). The twin epidemics of poverty and diabetes: Understanding diabetes disparities in a low-income Latino and immigrant neighborhood. *Journal of Community Health, 36*(6), 1032.

Diez-Roux, A. V., Nieto, F. J., Muntaner, C., Tyroler, H. A., Comstock, G. W., Shahar, E., ... & Szklo, M. (2017). Neighborhood environments and coronary heart disease: A multilevel analysis. *American Journal of Epidemiology, 185*(11), 1187–1202.

Downey, L. H. (2013). Rural populations and health: Determinants, disparities, and solutions. *Preventing Chronic Disease, 10*, E104. doi:10.5888/pcd10.130097.

Dover, D., & Belon, A. (2019). The health equity measurement framework: A comprehensive model to measure social inequities in health. *International Journal for Equity in Health, 18*(1), 36. doi:10.1186/s12939-019-0935-0.

Du Bois, W. E. B., & Eaton, I. (1899). The Philadelphia negro: A social study (No. 14). University of Pennsylvania Press.

Economic Research Service. (2018). Rural poverty & well-being. Retrieved from: www.ers.usda.gov/topics/rural-economy-population/rural-poverty-well-being/#geography.

Elliott, M. (2000). The stress process in neighborhood context. *Health & Place, 6*(4), 287–299.

Gee, G. C., & Ford, C. L. (2011). Structural racism and health inequities: Old issues, new directions. *Du Bois Review: Social Science Research on Race, 8*(1), 115–132. doi:10.1017/S1742058X11000130.

Gehlert, S., Mininger, C., Sohmer, D., & Berg, K. (2008). (Not so) gently down the stream: Choosing targets to ameliorate health disparities. *Health & Social Work, 33*(3), 163.

Gunderson, C., & Ziliak, J. (2015). Food insecurity and health outcomes. *Health Affairs, 34*(11), 1830–1839.

Hasan, M. K., Shahriar, A., & Jim, K. U. (2019). Water pollution in Bangladesh and its impact on public health. *Heliyon, 5*(8), e02145. Retrieved from: www.sciencedirect.com/science/article/pii/S2405844019358050.

Honjo, K. (2004). Social epidemiology: Definition, history, and research examples. *Environmental Health and Preventive Medicine, 9*(5), 193–199. doi:10.1007/BF02898100.

Kozyrskyj, A. L., Kendall, G. E., Jacoby, P., Sly, P. D., & Zubrick, S. R. (2010). Association between socioeconomic status and the development of asthma: Analyses of income trajectories. *American Journal of Public Health, 100*(3), 540–546.

Lahelma, E., Martikainen, P., Laaksonen, M., & Aittomäki, A. (2004). Pathways between socioeconomic determinants of health. *Journal of Epidemiology & Community Health, 58*(4), 327–332.

Marmot, M. (2005). Social determinants of health inequalities. *The Lancet, 365*(9464), 1099–1104.

McKinlay, J. B. (1979). A case for refocusing upstream: The political economy of illness. In J. Gartley (Ed.), *Patients, physicians and illness: A sourcebook in behavioral science and health* (pp. 9–25). New York, NY: Free Press.

National Academies of Sciences, Engineering, and Medicine. (2017). The state of health disparities in the United States. In *Communities in action: Pathways to health equity* (pp. 57–98). Washington, DC: The National Academies Press. Retrieved from: www.ncbi.nlm.nih.gov/books/NBK425844/.

National Center for Education Statistics. (2019). Public high school graduation rates: The condition of education. Retrieved from: https://nces.ed.gov/programs/coe/indicator_coi.a.

National Center for Health Statistics. (2018). *Health, US, 2017: With special feature on racial and ethnic health disparities*. Hyattsville, MD: National Centre for Health Statistics. Retrieved from: www.ncbi.nlm.nih.gov/books/NBK532685/.

National Congress of American Indians. (2019). *Tribal governance*. Available from: www.ncai.org/policy-issues/tribal-governance

National Research Council. (2004). Behavioral health interventions: What works and why? In *Critical perspectives on racial and ethnic differences in health in late life* (pp. 641–674). Washington, DC: The National Academies Press. Available from: www.ncbi.nlm.nih.gov/books/NBK25527/.

Neser, W. B., Tyroler, H. A., & Cassel, J. C. (1971). Social disorganization and stroke mortality in the black population of North Carolina. *American Journal of Epidemiology, 93*(3), 166–175. doi:10.1093/oxfordjournals.aje.a121243.

Office of Management and Budget. (2018). Race. Retrieved from: www.census.gov/topics/population/race/about.html.

Oreskovich, J. Z. H., & Zimmerman, H. (2012). Defining disability: A comparison of disability prevalence estimates produced by BRFSS and other data sources. Helena, MT: Department of Public Health and Human Services.

Powers, M., & Faden, R. (2006). *Social justice: The moral foundations of public health and health policy. Issues in biomedical ethics.* Oxford, UK: Oxford University Press.

Prevention Institute. (nd). Making the case fact sheet: Violence and health equity. Available from: www.preventioninstitute.org/sites/default/files/publications/Fact%20Sheet–Links%20Between%20Violence%20and%20Health%20Equity.pdf

Song, Z., & Baicker, K. (2019). Effect of a workplace wellness program on employee health and economic outcomes: A randomized clinical trial. *JAMA*, *321*(15), 1491–1501. doi:10.1001/jama.2019.3307.

Thomson, K., Hillier-Brown, F., Todd, A., McNamara, C., Huijts, T., & Bambra, C. (2018). The effects of public health policies on health inequalities in high-income countries: An umbrella review. *BMC Public Health*, *18*(1), 869. doi:10.1186/s12889-018-5677-1.

Tjaden, P., & Thoennes, N. (2000). *Full report of the prevalence, incidence, and consequences of intimate partner violence against women: Findings from the National Violence Against Women Survey.* Report prepared for the National Institute of Justice and the Centers for Disease Control and Prevention. Washington, DC: National Institute of Justice.

United Nations. (2014). Statistical annex development country classification. Retrieved from: www.un.org/en/development/desa/policy/wesp/wesp_current/2014wesp_country_classification.pdf.

Warnecke, R. B., Oh, A., Breen, N., Gehlert, S., Paskett, E., Tucker, K. L, ... & Hiatt, R. A. (2008). Approaching health disparities from a population perspective: The National Institutes of Health Centers for Population Health and Health Disparities. *American Journal of Public Health*, *98*(9), 1608–1615.

Wax-Thibodeaux, E. (2018). Here are 5 urgent problems a new VA secretary would need to tackle. *Washington Post.* Military. Retrieved from: www.washingtonpost.com/news/checkpoint/wp/2018/04/25/here-are-5-urgent-problems-a-new-va-secretary-would-need-to-tackle/.

Williams, D. R., & Sternthal, M. (2010). Understanding racial-ethnic disparities in health: Sociological contributions. *Journal of Health and Social Behavior*, *51*(Suppl.), S15–S27. doi:10.1177/0022146510383838.

Yen, I. H., & Kaplan, G. A. (1999). Neighborhood social environment and risk of death: Multilevel evidence from the Alameda County Study. *American Journal of Epidemiology*, *149*(10), 898–907.

3 Planning a social determinants of health focused evaluation

Learning objectives

After reading this chapter, you should be able to:

- Describe how to use SDOH in evaluation
- Summarize how to select a social determinant in the evaluation of public health programs
- Understand when SDOH focused evaluations are appropriate, and when they are not
- List differences between theories, frameworks, and paradigms
- Describe elements of a SDOH evaluation plan

Max was born November 22, 1919 during the Great Depression and the influenza pandemic. She was the fourth child out of five born in her family. Growing up in rural Kansas, she witnessed first-hand the effects of poverty, unemployment, limited housing, lack of health care, and limited social support. Her mother had inherited a small farm in western Kansas, but her parents were unable to make a living from it. Her father had a dray team of horses and hauled bricks to pave some city streets in rural Kansas. They had a milk cow, pigs, and chickens that provided some food for their family. Her mother sold eggs in town to earn money for the family. They moved every year, so Max went to a different school each year. Her extended family of cousins was large, providing some social support. This support was a tremendous strength throughout her life. At the end of eighth grade she worked and lived in a nearby city to save enough money so she could attend high school the following year.

At the time of her birth, and throughout the early years of her life, public health in the US was changing rapidly. State and local health authorities expanded their roles in the early 1900s to focus on health promotion rather than preventing disease. Leaders in public health envisioned that the twentieth century would bring scientific answers to disease, advanced medical treatment, and increased education about health habits that prolong life.

Fast forward 100 years. Today is November 22, 2019, and Max is 100 years old. She makes up one of the rare 1% of the US population that lives this long.

What was it about how Max lived that got her to 100? What were her social and environmental circumstances that supported this long life that few people experience? What is the role of public health in supporting life and longevity? Evaluation and the SDOH can help us answer these important questions.

On evaluation

There are two categories of SDOH program evaluation that we will focus on for the purposes of this chapter and SDOH, process and outcome evaluation. A **program** is a set of resources and activities directed toward one or more common goals (Newcomer, Hatry, & Wholey, 1994). **Program evaluation** is a systematic process of obtaining information to be used to assess and improve a program. Organizations and communities use program evaluations to distinguish successful program efforts from ineffective program activities and services. Results from evaluations can be used to revise existing programs to achieve successful results. Evaluations are a crucial part of any program. As you might recall from earlier chapters, process evaluations provide evidence that could improve the object of evaluation (or evaluand) and are generally cyclical in nature, documenting progress toward goals or objectives. In contrast, outcome evaluations help to create shared meaning about the evaluand and to support future decision making and are typically generated one time only, at the end of a program, policy, idea, or effort.

How to use SDOH in evaluation

By now you know the types of evaluation and when they are used in public health programs. You also have a broad understanding about the history of SDOH, examples of SDOH from the literature, and why they matter so much in evaluation. You might even feel excited about the potential of shifting evaluation efforts to focus on the underlying causes of health inequalities that can be linked to social determinants. But, how does this process happen? How can we shift evaluation approaches to encompass a focus on health equity and the SDOH? As we begin to conceptualize SDOH focused evaluations, we should consider these five questions (O'Neill & Simard, 2006):

1   Why evaluate?
2   What should be evaluated?
3   For whom is the evaluation produced?
4   Who is doing the evaluation?
5   How should the evaluation be conducted?

How might we answer these five questions? Let's begin with question one, **Why evaluate?** This might seem obvious for some, but not for all. There is an urgency in public health to create evidence-based programs and policies. Evaluation of public health programs and interventions builds evidence, tells funding agencies what to fund, and what not to fund, and grows scientific knowledge about the underlying causes of health inequalities in our world.

What should be evaluated? This depends largely on the goals of a program, policy, or intervention, and on what questions need to be answered. Take the example of health status. If the health status of a population is the focus, then what is the definition of health and what indicators will be used to measure health and changes over time? WHO-Europe identified 219 indicators to measure national scale progress toward 38 goals for Health for all Europe (WHO, 1989). This was too many and resulted in a failed evaluation of the impact of the Healthy Communities Movement in Europe (O'Neill & Simard, 2006).

For whom is the evaluation being produced? Is the evaluation required for a federal agency that funded the program? A local municipality? Community? Elected leaders? Faith-based organization? School? Academic institution and/or scientific body? Knowing answers to these questions before you undertake a SDOH focused evaluation is important because each requires a different level of information, more or less rigor, and varying levels of reporting and dissemination.

Who is doing the evaluation? There is a long history of who evaluates whom. Previous authors and communities discuss this in detail and share stories of power imbalances and struggles, oppressive systems, and deficit-focused, oppressive, and exploitative exercises. Transformative approaches in evaluation engage typically oppressed and marginalized groups, shifting power from evaluator or researcher to community or those populations that have been marginalized in the past.

How should the evaluation be conducted? What kinds of data are needed to conduct the evaluation? Answers to these questions largely depend on the focus of the evaluation, but one thing is known: SDOH focused evaluations utilize participatory and intersectoral approaches (Hancock, Labonte, & Edwards, 2000). Most often, these approaches take time to develop, because of gaining stakeholder buy-in, facilitating community review and approval, and asking for assistance with interpreting results. When multiple sectors are involved in an evaluation, at any level, this is expected, but it can take more time to reach consensus on various topics presented during the course of the evaluation.

In the next sections we will review what SDOH focused evaluation looks like in public health, and how you can incorporate four steps into the evaluation process. Let's begin with Step 1.

Step 1. Select a SDOH

The first step in developing a SDOH focused evaluation is to examine what the specific determinant or health outcome is that will be evaluated. Kaiser Permanente's Community Fund for the Social Determinants of Health outlines examples of SDOH goals and potential evaluation outcomes (Paige, Bourcier, Cahill, et al., 2012), as shown in Table 3.1.

Table 3.1 SDOH goals and definitions

Community cohesion
Grow social capital, improve cross-cultural understanding, build community,
   increase civic engagement.

Access to health care and disease prevention
Policy advocacy that expands health care access, culturally competent health
   workforce, and health promotion activities.

Food access and nutrition
Increase access to healthy foods through farmer's markets and healthy school
   lunch programs to address root causes of food insecurity.

Economic opportunities
Increase access to credit, job training programs, GED programs, and the
   development of co-ops.

Education and childhood development
Tutoring programs, pre-kindergarten programs, advocacy, school-based activities.

Housing
Access to housing and improved housing conditions.

Built environment, transportation, and environmental justice.
Access to active and reliable modes of transportation.
Local or regional planning with an equity and health lens.

Source: Adapted from Paige, Bourcier, Cahill, et al. (2012).

These SDOH goals are only examples. It is important to seek input from community advisory boards, partners, and colleagues to develop a SDOH focused evaluation—seek input early in the evaluation process.

Let's consider this example. Envision you are the evaluator for a city health department. You have been hired to evaluate the impact of a youth substance use prevention program. The goals of this program are to reduce binge drinking in youth by 30% and increase community readiness to address binge drinking by one overall point. The evaluation is focused on these two endpoints and measuring changes reported at the beginning of the program and five years later at the end of the program. Unfortunately, the evaluation is not focused on the underlying causes of substance abuse or environmental conditions that contribute to increases in binge drinking. Using a SDOH evaluation focus allows you to explore the determinants and approaches necessary to address these determinants.

To begin, review the literature to explore what determines substance abuse in youth. Use credible sources, community perspectives, published journal articles, and recent literature. A brief review of the published literature indicates that socioeconomic status, poor social support, family and social norms, crime, and hopelessness are key determinants of youth binge drinking (Galea, Nandi, & Vlahov, 2004). Sources also indicate that community conditions that increase youth binge drinking include lack of awareness about its dangers, easy access to alcohol, lack of enforcement in the community to address underage drinking, and limited prevention programs. With this information in mind, you can begin thinking about how an evaluation design could be used to explore these determinants. But first, it is a must to consider when SDOH focused evaluations are appropriate, and when they are not.

Step 2. Know when to use SDOH focused evaluations

Knowing when to use a SDOH focused evaluation is important because programs may not focus on an outcome that is linked to building health equity. For example, consider a case in which you were asked to evaluate a public health leaders' two-day conference. The evaluation contract outlined focus areas for the evaluation: satisfaction with the overall event, speakers, learning, reaction, and behavior change. This would not be an ideal SDOH focused evaluation opportunity because professionals at the event come from similar socioeconomic backgrounds, most have similar perspectives and training about public health, and the conference does not focus on health equity, structural inequalities, or the SDOH. Can you think of other examples when a SDOH focused evaluation might not be the best fit?

Below are some examples of when SDOH focused evaluations are appropriate (Metzler, nd).

- Policies and laws
- Violence
- Social gradient
- Social networks
- Culture and loss of culture, language, and traditions
- Transportation
- Racism and other forms of discrimination
- Aggregate characteristics of neighborhoods
- Physical living conditions
- Education
- Income
- Norms
- Social Support
- Social Capital
- Other areas that have been identified as important in addressing the underlying causes of a disease, disparity, health inequity, or inequality

Evaluations that focus on the SDOH are needed because there are limited health-specific prevention programs or research projects that examine SDOH in depth. Further, there has been limited research or evaluation conducted to determine the relationships between variables, or to develop a deeper understanding about interventions that could address the SDOH (Metzler, nd). This understanding is critical because much of what is known about PHE and SDOH is conceptual and, in most cases, not evidence based.

Step 3. Select a theory, know paradigms and frameworks

Understanding theories, models, frameworks, and paradigms used in SDOH focused evaluations will help you in the design process. The type of SDOH focused evaluation that you select should align with the program goals, culture, context, and needs.

A **theory** is a set of interrelated concepts, definitions, and ideas that generate a systematic view of events, situations, or relationships that help explain what is happening and why it is happening. A public health program may have an underlying program theory that outlines how a program is supposed to work. A **logic model** is often used in conjunction with a theory to visually outline relationships between programs, resources, processes, and intended outcomes. Logic models are based on program theories (see Appendix B for examples). **Models** are subclasses of theories and often draw on multiple theories rather than just one. Models are different from theories because they do not attempt to explain what is happening, just present information about the process.

There are a multitude of theories used in public health programs. One of the most common theories used in PHE is the theory of change. **Theory of change** describes what will happen as a result of a program and why. **Life course** theory involves exploring the complex ways that biological risks interact with economic, social, and psychological factors in the development of disease throughout one's life (Watt, 2002). Salutogenesis is a medical approach driven by factors that support human health and well-being rather than factors that cause disease. The **salutogenic model** (theory) focuses on identifying and modifying the sociostructural factors that influence the health status of populations. Examples include levels of education, working and housing conditions, and public-school quality and support—these salutary factors are thought to improve population health. **Social capital theory** involves exploring the psychosocial basis for health inequalities. Putnam (1993) defined social capital as the involvement in civic activities and organizations that creates norms of reciprocity, trust in mankind, that facilitate mutual benefits. Increased social support, social cohesion, and social networks may increase social capital and reduce health inequalities (Watt, 2002). **Ecosocial theory** blends social and physical environments and is the theory that lifestyle choices are influenced by life changes defined by where people live. **Psychosocial theories** may focus on discrimination and social hierarchy causing stress which then creates a neuroendocrine response that causes disease. The social product of health is another model that could be applied to a SDOH focused evaluation. Briefly, this is based on the idea that wealthy people gain material assets at a cost to the disadvantaged or resource poor communities. **Feminist theories** can be used to explore social justice, oppressive situations for women, gender domination, partial societies, objectification of women, invisibility, and exploration (Creswell & Poth, 2016). Critical theory and critical race theory are useful for comprehending, understanding, and transforming the underlying orders of social life and relationships that create community and society (Creswell & Poth, 2016). Critical race theory focuses on race and the racism that is embedded within societies and systems. **Queer theory** utilizes methods and strategies that bring to light an individual's identity and seeks to unpack gender as a binary concept. Queer theorists bring out voices of the oppressed through cultural engagement, advocacy, policy, and decon- struction of dominant theories (Sullivan, 2003). **Intersectionality theory** can help conceptualize a person, group of people, or social problem based on dis- crimination and disadvantage and multiple streams of oppression—for example, race, class, gender identity, sexual orientation, religion, and other identity markers (Hill Collins, 2019). There are more theories that could be applied to a SDOH evaluation, but it is important to move beyond the theoretical conceptual- izations about health inequalities and into models that can help us understand the social structure of health inequalities.

Models illuminate the importance of social structure in understanding causes of health inequalities, inequities, and injustice as they relate to the SDOH. It may seem like a lot, but if we know the theory, model, and paradigm, we can choose appropriate methods and frameworks to evaluate SDOH interventions. Later in this chapter we will explore how these theories guide frameworks that can be used to explore SDOH.

A brief note on paradigms versus frameworks and why the distinction matters may be useful. Paradigms are really about assumptions, philosophies, concepts, values, and a way of viewing reality. Paradigms may also be referred to as philo- sophical frameworks. A philosophical framework is used to determine how reality is explained, how knowledge is generated, and the perspective of the evaluator in research and practice (Monti & Tingen, 1999).

Paradigms

Paradigms are a basic set of beliefs that guide actions (Guba & Lincoln, 1998). An evaluator's paradigm is often based on a shared set of beliefs about how problems should be explored and addressed (Kuhn, 1970). Paradigms are often defined by ontology, epistemology, and methodology. Ontology is based on the question, "What is reality?" Epistemology is based on, "How do we know what we know?" And methodology is based on the question, "How will we go about collecting and gathering knowledge?" (Guba & Lincoln, 1998).

Evaluation paradigms are generally categorized as post-positivist, pragmatist, constructivist, advocacy/participatory, transformative, and materialist/structuralist. Briefly, a **post-positivist** evaluation is method driven. Method driven evalu- ations focus on what tools can be used to acquire knowledge. Typically, post- positivists design evaluations using quantitative evaluations, surveys, or experimental evaluation designs. The **pragmatist paradigm** is often focused on utility and usability—utilization focused evaluations are commonly pragmatist because the belief is that reality is constantly changing and unpredictable. A pragmatist evaluation often uses a mixed-method approach that is action based. **Constructivist** evaluations are value driven. These often include qualitative data, observation, narratives, and critical inquiry in the evaluation approach.

Transformative evaluation paradigms are based on the values of principles, equality, and justice (Guba & Lincoln, 1998). A **materialist/structuralist evaluation** approach might focus on low income levels that lead to a lack of resources, which in turn creates stress in life, and, eventually, poor health and disease.

One of the big questions that public health seeks to answer is how and why determinants cause disease or poor health? We can answer these big questions by utilizing the appropriate paradigm and methods.

Frameworks used in SDOH evaluations

Frameworks are based on the identification of key SDOH concepts or theories, and the relationships between them, and the evaluation goal. Frameworks can be philosophical, theoretical, or conceptual. The Canadian Council on Social Determinants of Health (2015) reviewed 36 frameworks on the SDOH. They report wide variation in frameworks used and their depiction of the SDOH. The Council's review resulted in six elements for consideration when developing a SDOH focused evaluation.

1   Use of a holistic approach
2   Use of an intersectoral approach
3   Recognition of social exclusion
4   Understanding of the role of individuals and communities
5   Recognizing of the importance of upstream action
6   Identification of interactions between determinants or feedback loops

In this chapter we will not review all 36, but it is imperative to know there are multiple frameworks that can be used in SDOH focused evaluations. Consider the Council's six elements listed above when selecting a framework.

For the purposes of this section on SDOH focused evaluation we will explore theoretical and conceptual frameworks. **Theoretical frameworks** are used to define variables in a SDOH evaluation. This may include designing evaluation questions, conducting the SDOH evaluation, analyzing data, understanding results, and applying results. **Conceptual frameworks** are useful for linking theory, themes, and findings of an evaluation. One of the common themes in SDOH frameworks is the presence of feedback loops, whereby determinants are influenced by multiple factors and multiple levels, with directionality of the loop changing based on a person's access to social position, the structure or information flow, and the strength of the feedbacks in relation to what is being targeted for intervention (Carey & Crammond, 2015).

SDOH are not new, but an evaluation approach that incorporates a SDOH focus is new for many public health professionals. If you are feeling overwhelmed with where to start, the DECIDE framework can help calm your nerves and get you on the right stream for SDOH focused evaluations. DECIDE is based on the following steps:

- Determine the SDOH goals the evaluation will address
- Explore specific SDOH questions that you will answer
- Choose the evaluation paradigm and techniques that you will use to answer evaluation questions
- Identify practical issues that you may encounter when implementing a SDOH focus
- Decide how you will deal with ethical issues that might come up
- Evaluate, interpret, and present SDOH evaluation findings

Participatory/collaborative evaluation frameworks are a good fit for SDOH focused evaluation. The DECIDE framework presented above emphasizes participatory/collaborative forms of evaluation, and engaging stakeholders, and gives voice to traditionally disadvantaged groups. This helps stakeholders understand evaluation and the program being evaluated and ultimately use the evaluation findings for decision-making purposes. As with utilization focused evaluation, the primary question guiding participatory evaluation is, "What are the information needs of those closest to the program?" These needs are then incorporated into the evaluation design and revisited throughout the evaluation process

Community-based participatory research (CBPR) is an approach that may also help guide SDOH evaluation planning efforts. CBPR is an approach to research based on collaboration, equity, and partnerships. It involves eight guiding principles, including: recognizing the community as a unit of identity, building on community strengths and resources, facilitating collaborative partnerships, integrating knowledge and action for mutual benefit, promoting co-learning and empowerment, employing cyclical and iterative processes, promoting health from strengths-based and ecological perspectives, and disseminating knowledge gained to all partners. CBPR approaches are most widely used in research involving health-related topics; however, they are beginning to emerge in other disciplines (Cargo & Mercer, 2008). CBPR is unique because it both values and promotes the strengths of communities to engineer social change (Israel, Coombe, Cheezum, et al., 2010). This approach should not be confused with **community engagement**, which is the application of institutional resources to address and solve challenges facing communities through collaboration with these communities (Saltmarsh, Giles, Ward, et.al, 2009).

WHO's SDOH framework combines psychosocial approaches, social production of disease/political economy of health, and ecosocial frameworks to understand the main pathways of health (Solar & Irwin, 2010). This framework is largely based on Diderichsen's model of the mechanics of health inequality (Diderichsen, Andersen, Manuel, et al., 2012). His model emphasizes social context, social stratification, differential exposure, differential vulnerability, and differential consequences of health. The SDOH framework is one of the most widely used in public health because it addresses multiple factors that impact

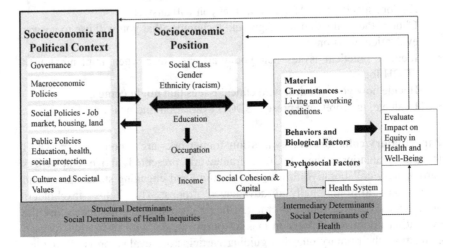

Figure 3.1 Social determinants of health framework.

Sources: Adapted from WHO (2008) and Solar & Irwin (2010).

equity in health and well-being. Here are some attributes of the framework, illustrated in Figure 3.1.

- Social–economic and political context include governance, macroeconomic policies, social policies, public policies, culture, and society's values.
- Socioeconomic position includes social class, gender, ethnicity (racism), education, occupation, and income. One's socioeconomic position is linked to social cohesion and social capital.
- Intermediary determinants of the SDOH are material circumstances, behaviors and biological factors, and psychosocial factors. These are influenced bidirectionally by the health system.
- Combined, these determinants impact equity, health, and well-being of populations.

Health impact pyramid

Health can be impacted at any point in time, but there are certain time points that are more effective for public health intervention than others. Frieden (2010) developed the **health impact pyramid** (shown in Figure 3.2) to illustrate the levels in which interventions could have the greatest impact. The base level of the pyramid includes the socioeconomic determinants, then public health interventions that change conditions for health, protective interventions that have long-term impact, clinical care, and counseling and education. His work indicates that intervention and programming that target the pyramid base (socioeconomic determinants), have the greatest potential to improve population health (Frieden, 2010).

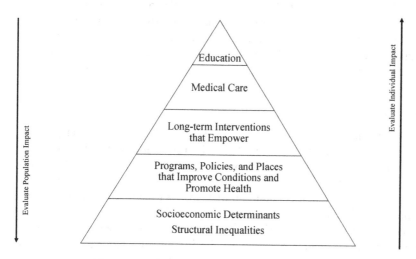

Figure 3.2 Health impact pyramid for SDOH focused evaluation.
Source: Adapted from Frieden (2010).

Risk and protective factors framework

Risk and protective factors include conditions that, when present, increase or decrease the likelihood of an adverse outcome (Piko, Fitzpatrick, & Wright, 2005). Risk and protective factors may be psychological, biological, or social. Factors may also be related to individuals, family, culture, community, or society. A SDOH focused evaluation that utilizes the risk and protective factors framework might explore risk factors such as limited family support, poverty, limited access to employment opportunities, domestic violence, crime involvement, substance abuse, and limited access to resources. Protective factors might include access to employment and quality education, access to quality health care, social support, and parental involvement and supervision. As you can see, the use of this framework will depend on the goals of the SDOH focused evaluation and the variables of interest.

Psychosocial approaches

Psychosocial approaches include factors that influence health, such as social networks, civic engagement, self-esteem, and hopefulness. SDOH evaluations rooted in a psychosocial framework focus on the following.

- Factors that mediate the effects of sociostructural factors on individual health outcomes
- Factors that are conditioned and modified by the social structures and contexts in which they exist (Martikainen, Bartley, & Lahelma, 2002)

Markwick and colleagues (2014) developed indicators of psychosocial risk factors that included food insecurity, psychological distress, and financial stress. Using a psychosocial framework, they found differences in Aboriginal and non-Aboriginal Victorians, where Aboriginal groups reported a higher prevalence of self-rated fair or poor health, cancer, asthma, and depression and anxiety.

Systems change frameworks

A focus on upstream factors that influence health is more effective than focusing on downstream factors. **Systems change frameworks**, therefore, are an important approach to consider when conceptualizing the SDOH evaluation. Systems change frameworks include organizations, systems issues, and how individuals/stakeholders/communities interact with these systems. An example of a systems change framework in SDOH is focusing on healthcare systems including general practice and health service organizations. Addressing public health problems like cancer, obesity, and substance abuse using a systems change framework lens can be more effective because the approach requires an examination of the entire system and how to produce change. Feedback loops are often used in systems change frameworks. An example from Carey and Crammond (2015) underscores the importance of feedback loops being balanced and reinforced. Taking their example, if the flu is left untreated, it creates reinforcing feedback loops: the more people who catch the flu, the more likely they are to infect others with the flu (Carey & Crammond, 2015). However, one of the major challenges with using systems change frameworks is that it is difficult to link desired changes to systems changes. This will be discussed along with other SDOH evaluation challenges in Chapter 4.

Health stigma and discrimination framework

The **health stigma and discrimination framework** recognizes that stigmatization is a process that occurs across the socioecological spectrum in the context of health (Stangl, Earnshaw, Logie, et al., 2019). These contexts vary across economic contexts in low-, middle-, and high-income countries. Domains in the framework include drivers and facilitators that impact health in affected populations, organizations, agencies, and communities across society.

Social–ecological model (SEM)

The **social–ecological model (SEM)** focuses on attitudinal variables at the intrapersonal level (McLeroy, Bibeau, Steckler, et al., 1988). SEM is a widely accepted model for use at the institution, community, policy, and intrapersonal levels (Kumar, Quinn, Kim, et al., 2011). Kumar and colleagues (2011) used the SEM, for example, to explore the 2009 H1N1 influenza vaccine uptake in the

US; this framework describes the factors that influenced evidence for determinants of the vaccine uptake, and the authors describe the SEM levels in detail. At the policy level, having health insurance or being in a priority group influenced uptake. At the community level, the presence of a disease or perceived risk increased uptake. At the institutional level, the availability of health care professionals and the information available within the organization influenced uptake. Interpersonal-level factors included the influence of social networks and the number of family and friends that received the vaccine. Finally, at the intrapersonal levels, there were several factors that influenced uptake. These included perceived risk from disease, perceived effectiveness, attitudes toward the vaccine, history of vaccine acceptance, perceived presence in a priority group, and trust of the government to handle the pandemic (Kumar et al., 2011). Figure 3.3 outlines the SEM levels, starting at the individual level, and text to the right links the SEM level to H1N1 vaccine uptakes. This example could be applied to multiple public health domains to target intervention points using a SDOH focus.

Life course framework (LCF)

Ben-Shlomo and Kuh (2002, p. 288, 291) write, "A life course approach is paradoxical as on the one hand it is intuitively obvious ... and yet on the other hand is empirically complex" and it "may help understand the underlying geographical patterns of mortality." The **life course framework (LCF)** recognizes that

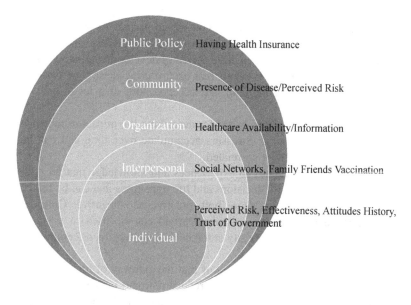

Figure 3.3 Social–ecological model with SDOH focus.

Source: Adapted from Kumar, Quinn, Kim, et al. (2011).

time and timing is important in documenting causal links between exposures and outcomes within people over the life course, across generations, communities, and populations (USDHHS, 2010). This framework is based on the life course theory (LCT), which is used to describe health and disease patterns across populations over time. LCT is useful in SDOH focused evaluation because it focuses on social, economic, and environmental factors that contribute to health disparities and health inequalities over time, population, and age groups.

WHO calls for use of the LCF to understand and promote the longevity revolution, and to document trends in health development and LCF factors that are associated with them, expanding the evidence base for what promotes health, and what takes away from it, and aligning the public health agenda with an LCF to support a global agenda for health equity (Caffe, 2017). Some of the features of the LCF that can help SDOH focused evaluations include the following:

- Pathways or trajectories that are built or depleted over a lifespan. We know that individual trajectories vary greatly but public health evaluators can assist in identifying patterns in populations and communities by examining the social, economic, and environmental factors that impact health (Caffe, 2017).
- Early programming—prenatal programming and intergenerational programming impact the health of the baby and mother.
- Cohorts, or a group of persons that share a common experience at a time in history, such as birth cohorts.
- Critical or sensitive periods which are considered periods of transition and time period of change. These include exposures or adverse events that impact a person at a critical or sensitive period of development. Pathways or trajectories are often driven by events that occur during these time periods, such as pregnancy, early childhood, adolescence, loss of a loved one, or retirement (Caffe, 2017).
- Cumulative impacts—these are useful for describing the impact of multiple stressors over the life course. Stressors accumulate over time and can be independent of one another or correlated.
- Transfer of assets. This relates to experiences and knowledge that an individual has that impact health decisions and life transitions that can be linked to multiple individuals. Assets are both positive and negative. Consider physical exercise and obesity. Lessons learned can be used to promote healthy lifestyles and reduce obesity at the individual, family, or community level.
- Risk and protective factors. These tell us that the pathway or trajectory that one is on can be changed. Actions that reduce risk and increase protective factors or resilience can help individuals and communities achieve health. Public health evaluators should consider the temporal relationship between determinants so that they can identify points for intervention. Risk and

protective factors are often used to explore what determines health and are often targets of change in SDOH focused evaluations (USDHHS, 2010).

Health equity measurement framework (HEMF)

The **health equity measurement framework** (HEMF) was developed by Dover and Belon (2019) to extend the SDOH causal frameworks to address health equity for ongoing public health surveillance and policy development.

This framework gained traction with the work of Yukiko Asada at the Department of Community Health and Epidemiology, Dalhousie University, and the Alberta Quality Matrix for Health.

Asada (2005) proposed a conceptual framework for health equity guided by three steps:

1   Define health distributions that are inequitable. This may include determinants of health, socioeconomic status, intervention points that modify human behaviors, and health overall.
2   Decide on measurement strategies to operationalize or define what equity would look like. What aspect of health will be measured? What is the unit of time under consideration? An entire lifetime, a point in time (cross-sectional), or a life stage approach?
3   Quantify health inequity information. Quantification may occur through comparisons, differences, aggregation, sensitivity to the mean, sensitive to the population size, and other subgroup considerations (Asada, 2005).

The **Alberta Quality Matrix for Health** has two components that influenced the HEMF: first, dimensions of quality such as patient and client experience; and, second, areas of need which focus services by the health system. Dover and Belon (2019), authors of the HEMF, note advantages in using HEMF rather than other SDOH frameworks. First, it encompasses multiple factors that affect health. Second, it describes the role of stakeholders and individuals in the process. The HEMF supports both cross-sectional and longitudinal evaluations and illustrates causal pathways between social determinants and health outcomes. The HEMF is the most recent, all-encompassing framework developed to target health inequities in populations across the world. Figure 3.4 is a conceptual model that outlines how to incorporate inequitable health distributions through SDOH focused interventions and evaluation.

A similar framework that takes into account health equity and systems thinking is the **equity-effectiveness loop framework**. This outlines five steps for developing or evaluating population health policies and programs, and is shown in Figure 3.5.

Community-driven solutions are foundational to building health equity. The "report framework," shown in Figure 3.6, is yet another example of how to address SDOH with a focus on structural inequities and biases, socioeconomic and political drivers (NAS, 2017).

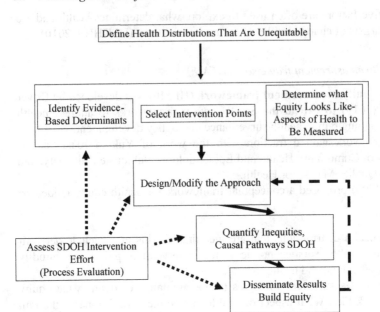

Figure 3.4 Health equity conceptual framework for SDOH evaluation.

Source: Adapted from Dover & Belon (2019).

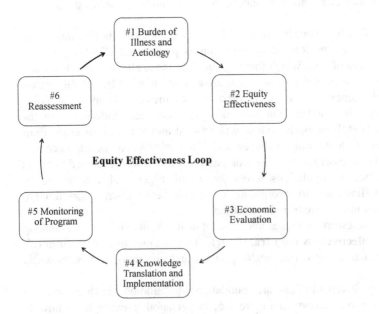

Figure 3.5 Equity-effectiveness loop.

Source: Adapted from Welch, Tugwell, & Morris (2008).

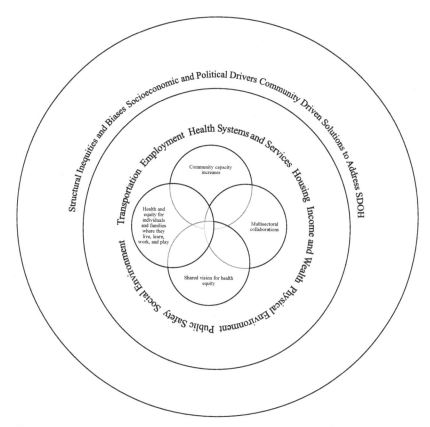

Figure 3.6 Report framework.

Source: Adapted from the National Academies of Sciences, Engineering, and Medicine (2017).

Step 4. Create a SDOH evaluation plan and implement it

The fourth step in a SDOH focused evaluation is to develop a plan and implement it. One common approach used in SDOH focused evaluation is the initiative planning model.

The initiative planning model (Timmreck, 2002) is similar to a logic model, but has a different focus. An initiative planning model can be used to illustrate your goals, objectives, action steps, and priorities. However, a key difference is that the initiative planning model focuses on a social determinant or specific outcome related to that determinant. This model also requires a review of evidence-based determinants in the literature, community definitions and perspectives of determinants, and approaches that could be used to address determinants. An example is illustrated in Figure 3.7.

Goal: To improve social determinants in order to reduce binge drinking in youth ages 12-20

Guiding Questions	Individual Objective:	Organizational Objective:	Community Objective:
What are the evidence-based determinants?	By 2020, increase awareness of social determinants of youth substance use	By 2021, increase the number and reach of substance use prevention programs	By 2022, increase number of youth enforcement officers in community
What other determinants are identified by the community?	**Approach:** Consciousness raising	**Approach:** Program development	**Approach:** Policy change
What will you do?	**Action Steps:** Create media campaign that educates policy makers, families, law enforcement, schools, and community members	**Action Steps:** Work with existing programs, policy leaders, and funders to expand prevention programming	**Action Steps:** Work with local officials to hire additional youth enforcement officers,
How long will it take? How much does it cost?			
What resources are needed?		**Resources & Costs:** Staff, grant funding or 3rd party billing for prevention, facilities, outreach efforts	**Resources & Costs:** Staff, grant funding or 3rd party billing for prevention, facilities, outreach efforts
How will you know if you have accomplished your goal?	**Resources & Costs:** Staff, media materials, billboard fees, web designer		

Figure 3.7 Initiative planning model to address youth binge drinking.

The planning model begins with answering key questions:

- What are the evidence-based determinants?
- What are other determinants identified by the community?
- What will you/the program do to address these determinants?
- How long will this take?
- How much will this program cost?
- What resources are needed?
- How will you know if you have accomplished your goals in addressing the social determinants?

As you can see, there are a lot of questions that evaluators need to ask to prepare for a SDOH focused evaluation. In some cases, there is an emerging evidence base about key determinants, but this evidence may not be reliable or confirmed. In these cases, seek community input to explore determinants of a given problem. Develop an evaluation that documents how these approaches impact the program goal. **Consider your community** and your stakeholders in the evaluation planning process. Is the topic important to them? Do they understand the issues and strategies to address the issue? What values guide community efforts? **Determine who your stakeholders are.** They might be the public, specific political stakeholders, or staff or program directors responsible for implementing a specific strategy. When planning with stakeholders consider their stake in the issue, who will benefit and who might lose. Will stakeholders support the policy or program? Who are the decision makers? (RWJF, 2019).

One of the key differences in a SDOH focused evaluation is that the focus is on changing the underlying conditions that contribute to a health disparity, inequality, or inequity rather than the outcome goal—in the example above the evaluation will report on whether the goal of reducing binge drinking by 30% was achieved, but that will not be the sole focus the evaluation. The primary focus of the SDOH evaluation of a binge drinking program is to determine if the approaches and action steps implemented had the intended effect on individual, organization, or community objectives (see Figure 3.7). This may sound a lot like a **process evaluation**, where evaluators document fidelity of a program through tracking attendance, participation, and exposure to enhance understanding about a program's impact (Steckler, Linnan, & Israel, 2002). While it is similar, a key difference is that the approach and action steps are designed based on the underlying determinants and the need to change these determinants. If, for example, you conducted a process evaluation on individual objective #1, to increase awareness of social determinants of youth substance use, this might include the number of youth and community members reached, the staff involved, the funding required, and contracts in place. In contrast a SDOH focused evaluation of individual objective #1 would focus on consciousness raising, and ask whether the program and action steps resulted in increased awareness of binge drinking among youth and how the action steps implemented led to these increases. Another difference in a SDOH focused evaluation might be an exploration of structural factors—for example, racial profiling and discriminatory practices of law enforcement against youth in certain neighborhoods or communities. There is a subtle difference, and this difference can mean everything in a SDOH focused evaluation.

Table 3.2 outlines potential areas for a SDOH focused evaluation of a prevention program to reduce youth binge drinking. Note that there are various levels at which the evaluation could be implemented, and nations, states, counties, communities, neighborhoods, and organizations may have different views about the indicators needed to conduct a SDOH focused evaluation.

We know that most programs are developed because there is a need. Often these needs are based on the disparities between two or more groups. Program examples include social service programs, violence prevention, public health programs, drug courts, intervention programs, health care quality and improvement programs, and more. Since most health inequalities can be rooted in social or economic conditions and structures, evaluators should consider a SDOH focused evaluation, even if it is not a requirement or explicitly stated in a program announcement.

One example of a federal program and funding that is based on a current need is the State Opioid Response program (SOR) by the Substance Abuse and Mental Health Services Administration (SAMHSA).

The Substance Abuse and Mental Health Services Administration (SAMHSA) is accepting applications for fiscal year (FY) 2018 State Opioid Response

Table 3.2 Youth binge drinking: potential areas for SDOH focused evaluation

SDOH Level	Health	Process		Impact	
		Process		*Impact*	
National State County Community Neighborhood Organization	Binge drinking individuals and populations	Access to prevention, education, community cohesion, fair policing	Youth and community engagement in prevention	Law enforcement racial profiling and discriminatory practices decrease	Goals achieved	Health and policy changes over time

Grants (Short Title: SOR). The program aims to address the opioid crisis by increasing access to medication-assisted treatment using the three FDA-approved medications for the treatment of opioid use disorder, reducing unmet treatment need, and reducing opioid overdose related deaths through the provision of prevention, treatment and recovery activities for opioid use disorder (OUD).

(SAMHSA, 2018)

The SOR focuses on the use of epidemiological data to demonstrate the critical gaps in availability of treatment for opioid use disorders (OUDs) in geographic, demographic, and service level terms; and to utilize evidence-based implementation strategies to identify which system design models will most rapidly and adequately address the gaps in systems of care. Under the evaluation criteria for this funding opportunity announcement (FOA), the only guidance is

Section E: Data Collection and Performance Measurement (approximately 1 page). Provide specific information about how you will collect the required data for this program and how such data will be utilized to manage, monitor and enhance the program.

(SAMHSA, 2018, p. 20)

Based on this guidance, evaluators could develop a SDOH focused evaluation, but it probably would not fit into their one-page requirements. And SDOH focused evaluation for the SOR would likely require a post-positivist paradigm that includes quantitative evaluations, surveys, or experimental evaluation designs. A brief review of evidence-based literature on the social determinants of OUD indicates that geography, race/ethnicity, and socioeconomic status are the primary factors that contribute to OUD in the US (Dasgupta, Beletsky, & Ciccarone, 2017). A SDOH focused evaluation could focus on improving the socioeconomic status of the target population through workforce development programs, education, job skills and readiness, general educational development (GED) programs, and policies that increase hiring of individuals with OUD.

Implement the plan

Once your SDOH evaluation plan is in place, it is time to implement the plan. Work with the community to identify areas that you will evaluate, assess needs and resources over time, act on what is important, and communicate information widely with community and stakeholders who have an interest in the SDOH focus area. Implementing a SDOH focused evaluation is similar to other evaluation approaches. The Robert Wood Johnson Foundation (2019) provides a clear step-by-step plan for implementing an evaluation plan.

- First, determine an organization's or community's readiness to conduct an evaluation and address the issue.

- Second, determine resources that are needed to support an evaluation. Typically, evaluations cost anywhere from 5% to 20% of a total budget. The amount of funding needed for an evaluation is dependent on a number of factors, such as the scope of the evaluation, the number of SDOH outcomes that will be assessed, the qualifications of the evaluator and their cost, and other resources available to the project.
- Third, identify core team members for the evaluation and make sure there is clarity around who will lead the evaluation and the responsibilities of each person (see Chapter 7 case study for guidance).
- Fourth, create a shared understanding about how the evaluation will be conducted and when evaluation results will be used. Earlier in this text we reviewed process, outcome, impact, or economic evaluation approaches.
- Fifth, identify benchmarks for success or milestones that track a program's success toward a goal.
- Sixth, implement the evaluation plan, use results to make program adjustments, inform policy, advocate for justice, or document benefits and impact on health disparities and inequalities. Report evaluation results for health equity (see Appendix A: Evaluation Report Outline).

Final thoughts on evaluation and SDOH

We started this chapter meeting Max, a 100-year-old who grew up during the Great Depression and the influenza pandemic. She experienced poverty, isolation, limited education, and unstable housing throughout her life, but these did not define her health. Why? I believe it is a mix of environmental conditions and context, behaviors that may be shaped by the environment, social grouping and status, and her biology. I do not have any data to support this, but I know from the WHO classifications of SDOH that these factors likely shaped her health. What needs to happen now? We need public health evaluations that explore the keys to longevity and quality of life for all people, of all racial and ethnic backgrounds, residences, occupations, religions, social capacities, or socioeconomic status.

We have covered a lot of ground in this chapter. By now you are familiar with the SDOH and how it can be used in evaluation. You also know the difference between a framework, a model, and a paradigm. We reviewed several examples of SDOH frameworks that could be used in SDOH evaluations. Know these and use these in your work.

Points to remember

When developing a SDOH focused evaluation, know that it is possible, and follow these four steps:

1   Select a social determinant of health.
2   Know when to use SDOH focused evaluations.

3   Select a paradigm and framework.
4   Create a SDOH evaluation plan and implement it.

If you are doing public health evaluation and using a SDOH focused approach, you are covering new ground. Prepare to be flexible, engage the community, and look at more than just the obvious determinants that impact public health. Engage community members in all steps of the evaluation process. People know what is happening in their communities and what is needed to address health inequalities, inequities, and disparities. Evaluation must address the root causes of disparities at the population level to impact the health of future generations.

Additional reading and resources

Life Course Perspective
Ben-Shlomo, Y., & Kuh, D. (2002). A life course approach to chronic disease epidemiology: Conceptual models, empirical challenges and interdisciplinary perspectives. *International Journal of Epidemiology*, 31, 285–293.

World Health Organization SDOH Framework
www.who.int/sdhconference/resources/ConceptualframeworkforactiononSDH_eng.pdf

Canadian Council's Review of Frameworks on the SDOH
http://ccsdh.ca/images/uploads/Frameworks_Report_English.pdf

Community Workbook
A community workbook for addressing the SDOH by Brennan Ramirez, L. K., Baker, E. A., & Metzler, M. (2008). *Promoting health equity: A resource to help communities address social determinants of health*. Retrieved from: www.cdc.gov/nccdphp/dch/programs/healthycommunitiesprogram/tools/pdf/SDOH-workbook.pdf

Chapter questions

1   Describe the four-step process for designing and implementing a SDOH focused evaluation. In your opinion, what is the most difficult step and why?
2   Review the SDOH goals in Table 3.1. List five additional SDOH goals that could be added to this table and defined using a SDOH lens.
3   Compare and contrast paradigms and frameworks that are used in the SDOH. Select a framework and apply it to a public health problem of interest.
4   Summarize four of the frameworks used in SDOH evaluation. Compare and contrast the benefits of each, and the limitations.
5   What is the DECIDE framework and how might this be helpful in planning a SDOH evaluation? What is this framework missing?
6   How might an evaluator identify evidence-based determinants for a public health program designed to prevent binge drinking in youth?

7   Create a conceptual model based on the youth binge drinking initiative planning model information. Use the socioecological model to guide your work and consider the public to individual levels (see Figure 3.3) to address binge drinking in youth.

Activities on the web

1   Conduct a brief literature review and identify a minimum of two additional frameworks that could be used in a SDOH focused evaluation. Provide a brief summary of the framework, the citation, and an example of how it was or could be used in a SDOH focused evaluation.
2   Type "paradigm" in a web search. Review three different definitions from separate websites. In your own words, describe your paradigm as an evaluator that incorporates SDOH.

References

Asada, Y. (2005). A framework for measuring health inequity. *Journal of Epidemiology & Community Health, 59*(8), 700–705.

Ben-Shlomo, Y., & Kuh, D. (2002). A life course approach to chronic disease epidemiology: Conceptual models, empirical challenges and interdisciplinary perspectives. *International Journal of Epidemiology, 31*(2), 285–293.

Caffe, S. (2017). *Social determinants of health and health inequalities: A life course approach.* 7th International Meeting on Indigenous Child Health. March 31, 2017.

Canadian Council on Social Determinants of Health. (2015). *A review of frameworks on the determinants of health.* Retrieved from: http://ccsdh.ca/images/uploads/Frameworks_Report_English.pdf.

Carey, G., & Crammond, B. (2015). Systems change for the social determinants of health. *BMC Public Health, 15*(1), 662. doi:10.1186/s12889-015-1979-8.

Cargo, M., & Mercer, L. (2008). The value and challenges of participatory research: Strengthening its practice. *Annual Review of Public Health, 29*, 325–350.

Creswell, J. W., & Poth, C. N. (2016). Qualitative inquiry and research design: Choosing among five approaches. Thousand Oaks, CA: Sage publications.

Dasgupta, N., Beletsky, L., & Ciccarone, D. (2018). Opioid crisis: No easy fix to its social and economic determinants. *American Journal of Public Health, 108*(2), 182–186.

Diderichsen, F., Andersen, I., Manuel, C., Andersen, A.-M. N., Bach, E., Baadsgaard, M., ... & Søgaard, J. (2012). Health inequality: Determinants and policies. *Scandinavian Journal of Public Health, 40*(8, Suppl.), 12–105. doi:10.1177/1403494812457734.

Dover, D., & Belon, A. (2019). The health equity measurement framework: A comprehensive model to measure social inequities in health. *International Journal for Equity in Health, 18*(1), 36. doi:10.1186/s12939-019-0935-0.

Frieden T. R. (2010). A framework for public health action: The health impact pyramid. *American Journal of Public Health, 100*(4), 590–595. doi:10.2105/AJPH.2009.185652.

Galea, S., Nandi, A., & Vlahov, D. (2004). The social epidemiology of substance use. *Epidemiologic Reviews, 26*(1), 36–52.

Guba, E. G., & Lincoln, Y. S. (1998). Paradigms in qualitative research. In Y. S. Lincoln & N. K. Denzin (Eds.), *The landscape of qualitative research: Theories and issues* (pp. 195–220). London, UK: Sage Publications.

Hancock, T., Labonte, R., & Edwards, R. (2000). *Indicators that count! Measuring population health at the community level.* Toronto, Canada: Centre for Health Promotion/ ParticipACTION.

Hill Collins, P. (2019). *Intersectionality as critical social theory.* Durham, NC: Duke University Press.

Israel, B. A., Coombe, C. M., Cheezum, R. R., Schulz, A. J., McGranaghan, R. J., Lichtenstein, R., ... & Burris, A. (2010). Community-based participatory research: A capacity-building approach for policy advocacy aimed at eliminating health disparities. *American Journal of Public Health, 100*(11), 2094–2102.

Kuhn, T. (1970). *The structure of scientific revolutions* (2nd ed.) (pp. 31–65). Chicago, IL: University of Chicago Press.

Kumar, S., Quinn, S. C., Kim, K. H., Musa, D., Hilyard, K. M., & Freimuth, V. S. (2011). The social ecological model as a framework for determinants of 2009 H1N1 influenza vaccine uptake in the United States. *Health Education & Behavior, 39*(2), 229–243.

Markwick, A., Ansari, Z., Sullivan, M., Parsons, L., & McNeil, J. (2014). Inequalities in the social determinants of health of Aboriginal and Torres Strait Islander people: A cross-sectional population-based study in the Australian state of Victoria. *International Journal for Equity in Health, 13*(1), 91. doi:10.1186/s12939-014-0091-5.

Martikainen, P., Bartley, M., & Lahelma, E. (2002). Psychosocial determinants of health in social epidemiology. *International Journal of Epidemiology, 31*(6), 1091–1093. doi:10.1093/ije/31.6.1091.

McLeroy, K. R., Bibeau, D., Steckler, A., & Glanz, K. (1988). An ecological perspective on health promotion programs. *Health Education Quarterly, 15*(4), 351–377.

Metzler, M. (nd). Social determinants of health information sheet: Community based participatory action research activity. Centers for Disease Control and Prevention, Division of Prevention Research and Analytic Methods. Retrieved from: www.orau.gov/cdcynergy/soc2web/Content/activeinformation/resources/SOC_SDOH_%20Fact_Sheet_112001.pdf.

Monti, E. J., & Tingen, M. S. (1999). Multiple paradigms of nursing science. *Advances in Nursing Science, 21*(4), 64–80.

National Academies of Sciences, Engineering, and Medicine. (2017). The root causes of health inequity. In *Communities in action: Pathways to health equity* (pp. 99–184). Washington, DC: The National Academies Press. Available from: www.ncbi.nlm.nih.gov/books/NBK425845/.

Newcomer, K. E., Hatry, H. P., & Wholey, J. S. (1994). *Meeting the need for practical evaluation approaches: An introduction. Handbook of practical program evaluation.* San Francisco, CA: Jossey-Bass Inc.

O'Neill, M., & Simard, P. (2006). Choosing indicators to evaluate Healthy Cities projects: A political task? *Health Promotion International, 21*(2), 145–152.

Paige, S., Bourcier, E., Cahill, C., Hsu, C., & Kabel, C. (2012). Evaluating the Kaiser Permanente community fund's social determinants of health portfolio. *The Foundation Review, 4*(1). doi:10.4087/FOUNDATIONREVIEW-D-11-00030.

Piko, B. F., Fitzpatrick, K. M., & Wright, D. R. (2005). A risk and protective factors framework for understanding youth's externalizing problem behavior in two different cultural settings. *European Child & Adolescent Psychiatry, 14*(2), 95–103.

Putnam, R. (1993). *Making democracy work: Civic traditions in modern Italy* (p. 63). Princeton, NJ: Princeton University Press.

Robert Wood Johnson Foundation. (2019). County health rankings key activities. Retrieved from: www.countyhealthrankings.org/key-activities/18391#key-activity-6.

Saltmarsh, J., Giles, D. E., Ward, E., & Buglione, S. M. (2009). Rewarding community-engaged scholarship. *New Directions for Higher Education*, (147), 25–35.

Solar, O., & Irwin, A (2010). *A conceptual framework for action on the social determinants of health*. Social Determinants of Health Discussion Paper 2 (Policy and Practice). World Health Organization. Retrieved from: https://apps.who.int/iris/bitstream/handle/10665/44489/9789241500852_eng.pdf.

Stangl, A. L., Earnshaw, V. A., Logie, C. H., van Brakel, W., Simbayi, L. C., Barré, I., & Dovidio, J. F. (2019). The Health Stigma and Discrimination Framework: A global, crosscutting framework to inform research, intervention development, and policy on health-related stigmas. *BMC Medicine 17*, 31. doi:10.1186/s12916-019-1271-3.

Steckler, A. B., Linnan, L., & Israel, B. (2002). *Process evaluation for public health interventions and research* (pp. 1–23). San Francisco, CA: Jossey-Bass.

Substance Abuse and Mental Health Services Administration. (2018). State Opioid Response Funding Announcement. CFDA 92.788. Retrieved from:www.samhsa.gov/grants/grant-announcements/ti-18-015.

Sullivan, N. (2003). *A critical introduction to queer theory*. New York, NY: NYU Press.

Timmreck, T. (2002). *Planning, program development, and evaluation: A handbook for health promotion, aging and health services*. Sudbury, MA: Jones & Bartlett.

US Department of Health and Human Services. (2010). *Rethinking MCH: The life course model as an organizing framework. Concept paper*. Retrieved from: www.hrsa.gov/sites/default/files/ourstories/mchb75th/images/rethinkingmch.pdf.

Watt, R. G. (2002). Emerging theories into the social determinants of health: Implications for oral health promotion. *Community Dentistry and Oral Epidemiology*, *30*(4), 241–247.

Welch, V., Tugwell, P., & Morris, E. B. (2008). The equity-effectiveness loop as a tool for evaluating population health interventions. *Revista de Salud Pública*, *10*, 83–96.

World Health Organization. (1989). Revised list of indicators and procedure for monitoring progress towards Health for All in the European region (1987–1988). Copenhagen, Denmark: WHO European Bureau.

World Health Organization. (2008). *Closing the gap in a generation: Health equity through action on the social determinants of health, final report*. Geneva, Switzerland: WHO Commission on Social Determinants of Health.

4 Collecting and analyzing SDOH data

Learning objectives

After reading this chapter, you should be able to:

- Define quantitative and qualitative data
- List four challenges of conducting a SDOH focused evaluation
- List two examples of population health solutions
- Compare and contrast surveys, scales, questionnaires, and indices
- Explain data sources available for SDOH focused evaluations and why they are appropriate to use
- Differentiate SDOH considerations in the United States and developing countries

We have covered a lot of ground in the last three chapters. By now you know the history of SDOH, upstream, midstream and downstream approaches, and the steps for planning SDOH focused evaluation in PHE. Before we begin reading about data collection, and the challenges and solutions of SDOH focused evaluations, I must share this with you—the SDOH vary by country and condition. Although we have read about SDOH based on a global perspective in the previous chapters, we must recognize that SDOH are unique to country and condition as well. This means there is not a one size fits all approach to conducting SDOH evaluations, so flexibility and place-based evaluation models are needed to rise to the challenge and actually implement effective SDOH programming and evaluations.

There is no necessary biological reason why life expectancy should be 48 years longer in Japan than in Sierra Leone or 20 years shorter in Australian Aboriginal and Torres Strait Islander peoples than in other Australians. Reducing these social inequalities in health, and thus meeting human needs, is an issue of social justice (Marmot, 2005, p. 8).

Let's start by looking at the importance of data.

Collecting SDOH data

Linking SDOH data to health outcomes can be a major challenge. There is agreement in the United States that there is a need for improved conceptualization and access to data that support a SDOH evaluation focus on how the social environment impacts the health of populations (Marmot, 2005). But what is data and what does it look like in SDOH evaluation?

Often the terms primary and secondary data sources are used to describe data sources. **Primary data** collection sources include surveys, interviews, focus groups, document reviews, meeting minutes, and more. **Secondary data** sources are those which already exist. In SDOH evaluations secondary data sources include US Census data, state vital statistics, various national and state surveillance databases, US Department of Agriculture (USDA) Economic Research Service data, US Environmental Protection data, National Center for Education Statistics data, and more. **Administrative data** is another type of secondary data that may be collected by an organization or business. Some examples of administrative data include hospital intake and discharge records, employee records, police records, daily sales, and others. The use of primary or secondary data sources in evaluation depends on a number of different factors. Using primary data may be preferred because evaluation instruments can be designed to answer questions relating to a specific SDOH focus area. The downside of primary data collection is the expense of collecting data—this often requires travel to the community, preparing instruments, collecting the data, and analyzing the data. Using secondary data is often preferred because it does not require any data collection on your part, and it is inexpensive—most secondary data sets are available online.

Typically, data is characterized as qualitative or quantitative. **Quantitative data** collection methods include any method that results in a response that is or can be transformed into a number. Quantitative data answers question like "How many?", "Who was involved?", "What was the outcome?", "How much did it cost?", and "What changed?" **Qualitative data** methods answer questions like "What is the value?", "What happened?", "How did people feel?" (Agency for Toxic Substances Disease Registry [ATSDR], 2015). Qualitative data may be collected via forms, surveys, or questionnaires using open text response. A **survey** is used to collect data from individuals that is mainly closed ended. In some cases, open text responses may be used to further explore individual ideas, beliefs, or behaviors regarding a specific topic. **Focus groups** are a discussion among a group of people about a specific issue. **Interviews** are a form of qualitative data used to document perspectives, experiences, and ideas about a given project or context. **Structured interviews** are typically used when responses are established already, and respondents select from a list of pre-established answers rather than open-ended questions. Questions are asked in a specific order and the approach is focused and rigid. **Semi-structured interviews** are often developed based on a guiding theme or principle that is underpinning a SDOH evaluation. **Unstructured interviews** are discussions about what is happening and are not based on a theme or set of questions. An **evaluation instrument** is anything that is used to collect the information that is needed in the evaluation. A **questionnaire** is a set of questions in a survey that includes qualitative and quantitative questions. Questionnaires may be used to document behavior, facts, or preferences—these can be incorporated into a scale. A **scale** includes multiple items that are related to one another. Likert-type scales are often used to assess levels of agreement regarding a specific topic, such as housing discrimination. An **index** is like a scale but different in that the goal is to calculate an index score for a series of statements or questions (that are indicators) related to a specific line of inquiry. For example, an evaluator might use an index to explore well-being using three questions designed to measure subjective well-being and having yes or no responses. Index scores are then calculated based on the number of yes responses and that number is their score. Sometimes the terms indicator, metric, or measure are used interchangeably to mean the same thing, so before you begin an evaluation, make sure you are using the correct terms. Other types of measures include targets, benchmarks, or standards. The US Agency for International Development (US AID, 2010) defines performance indicators as a measure of change that demonstrates if goals and objectives were achieved. Here are some types of indicators that US AID identifies as important in evaluation.

- Performance indicators provide information and evidence that change is occurring
- Standards indicators are often used in reporting to measure change in laws, policy, or regulatory practices
- Contextual indicators help understand social and environmental conditions that impact programs and populations—an example is a social vulnerability index score

Data challenges

Data sources and collection may also include news and internet, observation, funding agency reports, grant proposals, and other data sources needed to explore SDOH in evaluation. While there are multiple data sources and tools available, there are challenges that you must be aware of before you begin. First, the nature of self-reported data related to social or economic conditions means that it may not be provided, or, in some cases, be accurate. Lofters and colleagues report that people are uncomfortable disclosing household income, particularly in healthcare settings (Lofters, Shankardass, Kirst, et al., 2011). Second, there may be large amounts of missing data, due to the reasons just described or other factors. Third, approval for collecting such data may be difficult to achieve; for example, with Indigenous persons there are unique ownership, control, and access principles that must be adhered to (Lofters, Schuler, Slater, et al., 2017). Language and how questions are asked may result in difficulty in comparing data between persons and countries. It may be difficult to collect enough SDOH data that is representative of a community or population. These data challenges are not insurmountable, and selection of a transformative paradigm with advocacy and participatory planning and data collection methods can help ensure that SDOH data is on target, represents the needs of the community and underrepresented groups, and involves shared power. Consider who is at the table and who should be at the table as you think about data.

Finding data

Although finding SDOH data can be difficult, it is not impossible. There are resources available that can support a SDOH focused evaluation. Hillemeier and colleagues at the National Center for Chronic Disease Prevention and Health Promotion (Hillemeier, Lynch, Harper, et al., 2004) developed a directory for SDOH variables that could be used in a SDOH focused evaluation. They characterized 12 dimensions of the social environment and identified multiple data sources. **Economic components** include income, wealth, poverty, economic development, financial services, cost of living, redistribution, fiscal capacity, and exploitation. For each of these components, multiple indicators and data sources are available. **Employment components** include employment and unemployment rates, workforce characteristics, area business capacity, job access, occupational safety, job quality, and job characteristics. **Education components** include educational attainment, funding, private schools, school characteristics, and community climate. **Political components** include civic participation, political structure, and power groups. Power groups refers to the number of community organizations or unions and to their size and involvement in civic, social, human rights, environmental, and business endeavors in a community. **Environmental components** include air quality, water quality, environmental hazards, physical safety, and land use. Examples of physical safety include traffic and needed street repairs. **Housing components** include housing stock, residential patterns, regulation, and financial issues. Examples of residential patterns include homelessness, number of institutional facilities, segregation, vacancy rates, crowed housing, and population density. **Medical components** include primary care, specialty care, emergency services, home health care services, mental health care, long-term care, oral health care, and access to and utilization of care. **Governmental components** include funding, policy and legislation, services, and municipal fragmentation. An example of municipal fragmentation might be the number of local government and metropolitan power diffusion indices. **Public health components** include programs, regulations and enforcement, and funding. **Psychosocial components** include political activity, volunteer organizations, union participation, charitable giving, jails, lawsuits, and protective services. **Behavioral components** include tobacco use, physical activity, diet and obesity, alcohol and illicit drug use, and violence. **Transport components** include safety, infrastructure, traffic patterns, vehicles, public transportation, and economic issues.

One aspect of SDOH evaluation that you will need to decide early in the planning process is the kinds of data that you have available based on the evidence-based determinants identified in your review of literature and on discussions with community and other stakeholders. In the United States, there are a number of data sets available that match each of the 12 dimensions of the social environment mentioned previously. In the next section we will explore selected components and data sources that could be used for SDOH focused evaluations.

Income distribution. Higher levels of economic resources (income in this case) are directly related to more optimal health (Krieger, Chen, Waterman, et al., 2002). One way to measure income distribution and economic inequality is the **Gini index**, also called the Gini coefficient. Named for Italian statistician Corrado Gini in 1912, the Gini index ranges from 0 to 100% with 0 representing complete equality and 100 representing complete inequality (Chappelow, 2019). Consider a country where everyone has an income of $30,000 per year. In this country, the Gini index is 0. In contrast, in a country where one person earned all the income possible, let's say $1,000,000 and other residents of that country earned $0, the Gini index would be 1. Check out Figure 4.1, which compares Gini indices for US households by race from 2008 to 2018.

Employment. Unemployment rates and occupational status are often used as indicators of deprivation and associated with poorer health. Data from the Bureau of Labor and Statistics provides information on employment status for the civilian labor force by race/ethnicity, state, gender, and household status. Figure 4.2 outlines unemployment rates by race and Latino ethnicity. 2018 data shows that African American men in Alabama have the highest rates of unemployment in the state, at 7.4% of the population. In contrast, the lowest unemployment rates are among married men with a spouse present, at just 1.5%

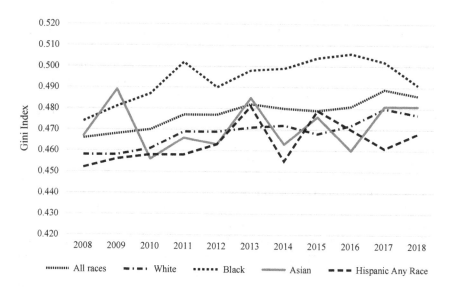

Figure 4.1 Gini index income disparity by race and origin of households 2008–2018.

Source: US Bureau of the Census, Current Population Survey, Annual Social and Economic Supplements (2019). Retrieved from: www.census.gov/data/tables/time-series/demo/income-poverty/historical-income-inequality.html.

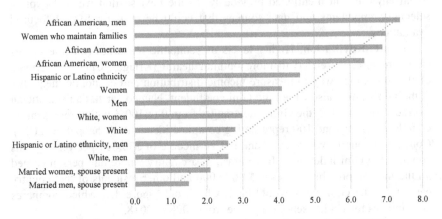

Figure 4.2 Alabama average unemployment rate by race, Latino ethnicity 2018.

Source: Bureau of Labor Statistics (2018). Expanded State Employment Status Demographic Data. Retrieved from: www.bls.gov/lau/ex14tables.htm.

of the population. Data shows that one's race and ethnicity can be associated with higher unemployment rates.

Education. Funding for education has a direct impact on educational attainment and is a solid predictor of school characteristics and community/political support for education. Data from the National Center for Education Statistics (NCES) shows disparities in state revenue per pupil, Figure 4.3 shows differences in revenues per pupil by state, with the highest funding allocated to the District of Columbia and the lowest to Idaho. If we examine average freshman graduation rates for White students living in both of these states, the graduation rate is 87.8% in the District of Columbia and 85% in Idaho (NCES, 2019). SDOH focused evaluations in education can drive policies and investments such as equitable school funding, universal pre-k programs, college scholarships, and cradle to career programs so that all youth receive the education they need to be successful (National Equity Atlas, 2019).

Education and poverty are inextricably linked. Data from the American Housing Survey shows a graded relationship between the level of education achieved (graduate to less than ninth grade) and poverty level and food stamp eligibility. This is illustrated in Figure 4.4.

Political components. The percentage of women elected to statewide offices is one way to document the political structure of a state or county. Data from the Center for American Women and Politics (CAWP) (www.cawp.rutgers.edu) reports that in 2019 there were 126 women in Congress, making up 23.6% of all 535 seats. Ninety-one women hold statewide elective executive offices in the US, making up 29.3% of all available positions for governors and lieutenant governors. Women are mayors in 27 of the 100 of largest US cities (CAWP, 2019). The US Census provides state and local government expenditures by year and category. Funding for health-related programs directly relates to conditions

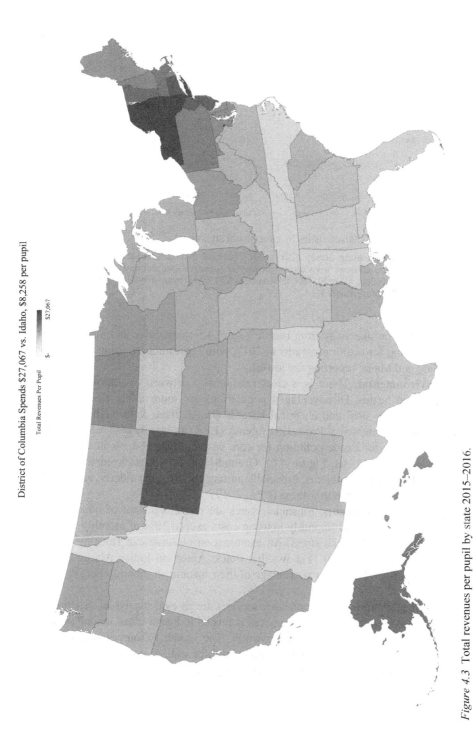

Figure 4.3 Total revenues per pupil by state 2015–2016.

Source: National Center for Education Statistics (2019). State Revenue Per Pupil by Source.2015–2016. Retrieved from: https://nces.ed.gov/ccd/elsi/expressTables.aspx.

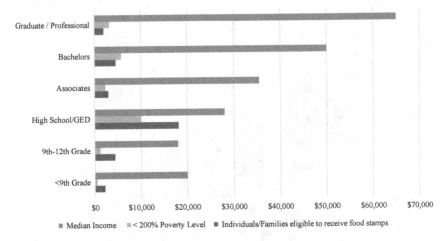

Figure 4.4 Income characteristics by educational attainment.

Source: American Housing Survey (2019). 2017 National Income Characteristics Education of Householder. Retrieved from: www.census.gov/programs-surveys/ahs/data/interactive/ahstablecreator. html?s_areas=00000&s_year=2017&s_tablename=TABLE9&s_bygroup1=20&s_bygroup2=14&s_filtergroup1=3&s_filtergroup2=1.

that support or take away from health. Figure 4.5 shows state and local government funding for health programs in 2017, with California reporting the highest funding and Maine reporting the lowest.

Environmental. There is a clear relationship between environmental conditions and health. Disadvantaged populations are more likely to experience exposure to physical and chemical hazards (Hajat, Hsia, & O'Neill, 2015). A review of Environmental Protection Agency (EPA) air quality data reports eight-hour averages for ozone pollution for core based statistical areas in the United States (EPA, 2019; see Figure 4.6). Ground-level ozone has been linked to a multitude of health problems, especially among children, the elderly, and people with lung diseases such as asthma (EPA, 2019).

Housing components. Financial issues are one component of housing that relate to SDOH. When monthly housing costs exceed 30% of monthly income, this may create financial stress. An examination of American Housing Survey data (as given in Table 4.1) shows that Black, American Indian Alaska Native, and Asians spend a greater percentage of their income on monthly housing than Whites.

Medical components. Health care services are an evidence-based determinant of health. Access to health care services is related to health status among populations in the US and throughout the world. The Health Resources and Services Administration (HRSA) tracks the health workforce and geographic areas based on medically underserved populations and health professional shortage areas (HPSAs). Areas with the most extreme need for health professionals in primary care, dental

State and Local Government Funding for Health Programs by State 2017: California
Highest- $23,037,657 and Maine is the Lowest- $190,515

State and Federal Funding

$23,037,657

$190,515

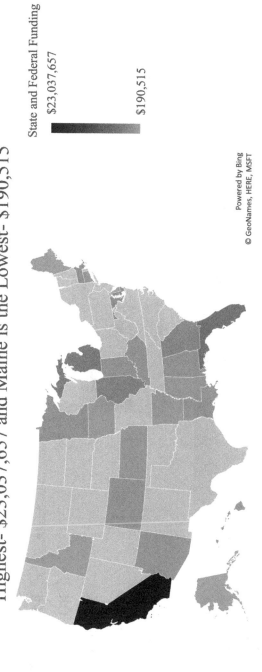
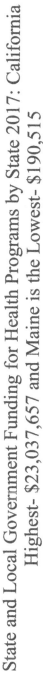

Powered by Bing
© GeoNames, HERE, MSFT

Figure 4.5 State and local government funding for health programs by state 2017.

Source: US Census Bureau (2019). 2017 State and Local Government Finance Historical Datasets and Tables. Retrieved from: www.census.gov/data/datasets/2017/econ/local/public-use-datasets.html.

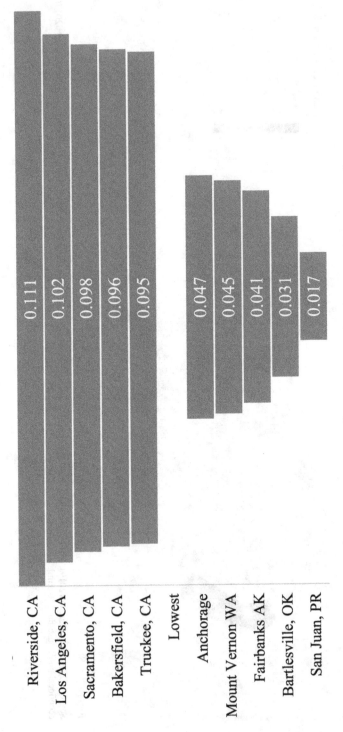

Figure 4.6 Ground-level ozone concentrations by statistical area.

Source: Environmental Protection Agency (2019). Air Quality Statistics by City, 2018. Ozone 8-hour average parts per million. Retrieved from: www.epa.gov/ground-level-ozone-pollution.

Table 4.1 Housing cost as a percentage of household income by race

Percentage of Income Spent on Housing	Total Estimate	White	Black	AIAN	Asian
Median Percent	21%	20%	25%	23%	23%
	Total Estimate	White	Black	AIAN	Asian
35–39%	6,214	4,581	1,021	106	400
40–49%	7,537	5,667	1,213	119	254
50–59%	4,676	3,389	846	61	151
60–69%	2,768	1,961	573	S	213
70–99%	4,295	3,138	785	59	388
100%	8,024	5,776	1,644	81	185

Source: American Housing Survey (2019). 2017 National Income Characteristics Education of Householder. Retrieved from: www.census.gov/programs-surveys/ahs/data/interactive/ahstablecreator. html?s_areas=00000&s_year=2017&s_tablename=TABLE10&s_bygroup1=20&s_bygroup2=9&s_filtergroup1=1&s_filtergroup2=1.

Note: AIAN = American Indian Alaska Native.

health, and mental health are low-income populations, followed by Medicaid populations, other/low-income migrant farmworker populations, correctional facilities (inmates), homeless populations, and tribal/rural areas (HRSA, 2019).

Psychosocial components. Social interactions and relationships create social capital. Social capital drives trust, norms, and networks, and improves society. Psychosocial dimensions that determine health include trust, fairness, helpfulness, crime or collective well-being, and civic engagement (Hillemeier et al., 2004). Let's consider crime as an indicator of collective well-being that is influenced by social capital. Data from the Bureau of Justice Statistics (BJS) shows that there were 1,489,363 people in US prisons at the end of 2017 (BJS, 2019). Black females were twice as likely as White females to be placed in state or local prisons (92 per 100,000 vs. 49 per 100,000), while the Hispanic imprisonment rate was 66 per 100,000 during this same time period. More than half of the offenders in federal prisons were in prison for drug-trafficking offenses. Violent crimes accounted for a large number of sentences as well, with 60% of Hispanics and Blacks in state prison being sentenced for violence compared with 48% of White prisoners. Reports from the Bureau of Justice show that Black males were six times more likely than White males to be imprisoned (2,336 per 100,000 vs. 397 per 100,000) (BJS, 2019).

Behavioral components. Determinants of premature morbidity and mortality include tobacco use, physical activity, diet and obesity, alcohol and illicit drug use, and violence. Exposure to violence is an evidence-based determinant of health. Data from the Behavioral Risk Factor Surveillance System (www.cdc.gov/brfss) includes prevalence data for a number of these determinants. Let's explore rates of violent crime in the US. Data from the Federal Bureau of Investigation indicates that in 2018, there were 380.6 violent crimes per 100,000 population, this is a significant decrease from 2008 when the rate was 458.6 per 100,000.

Transport components. Transportation directly impacts health. While motor vehicle deaths are the number one cause of injury in the United States, there are other aspects of transportation that impact health. Being able to maintain a job/ employment or access medical care are often determined by having access to reliable transportation. The number of vehicles per household impacts how individuals get to and from work, health care, and their ability to engage in activities that promote health (faith-based organizations, civic engagement, volunteerism, physical and recreational activities). American Community Survey (ACS) data indicates that 8.8% of households do not have a vehicle available, 33.2% have one vehicle, and 37.4% have two vehicles available (ACS, 2017).

US data sources

American Community Survey (ACS). If you live in the United States, you are probably aware of the ACS. ACS collects information annually on jobs, educational attainment, housing status, health care access, transportation, and other SDOH domains. Much of our focus in this text has been on education, income, and housing. What can we learn about SDOH from existing data that comes from the ACS? I live in New Mexico and would like to know more about educational attainment, income, and poverty in my state. A quick tap on ACS quick facts takes me to New Mexico, where I can see the median household income is $46,718, 21% of individuals live below the poverty level, the median age is 37.3 years, and 85% are high school graduates or higher (ACS, 2019). New Mexico ACS data (2019) provides information on housing and transportation, where 67% of homes are owner occupied and 6% of houses do not have a car or transportation available.

The **Centers for Disease Control and Prevention (CDC).** If you need SDOH data, CDC may have it. Some of the most frequently used population health surveys include the **Behavioral Risk Factors Surveillance System (BRFSS).** BRFSS is the largest continuously conducted health survey system in the world, conducting telephone interviews with more than 400,000 US adults each year in all 50 states, the District of Columbia, and several US territories. The **National Health and Nutrition Examination Survey (NHANES)** is a program that explores health and nutritional characteristics of adults and children throughout the United States. Beginning in 1960, NHANES has continuously led the nation in sampling 5,000 persons each year across the country to track demographic, socioeconomic dietary, and health-related questions. The **Youth Risk Behavior Survey (YRBS)** is part of the CDC's Youth Risk Behavioral Surveillance System (YRBSS) that monitors health behaviors among high school students from across the United States. Other CDC surveys that can help SDOH focused evaluations include the National Health Interview Survey, National Health Care Survey Registry, National Immunization Survey, National Survey of Family Growth, National Ambulatory Medical Care Survey, National Hospital Discharge Survey, National Medical Expenditure Survey, National Nursing Home Survey, and National Survey of Ambulatory Surgery. These and other data sets encompass economy, employment, education, political, environmental, housing, medical, public health, psychosocial, behavioral, and transport dimensions (see: www.cdc.gov/dhdsp/docs/data_set_directory.pdf, for a directory of available data sets).

Gallup-Healthways Well-Being Index (WBI) is a compilation of three million surveys completed by people in the United States and around the world (https://wellbeingindex.sharecare.com/). The WBI explores well-being in communities, states, and populations using clinical research, health care leadership, and behavioral economics. Aspects of well-being in the index include purpose, and social, financial, community, and physical well-being.

The **Bay Area Regional Health Inequities Initiative (BARHII)** is a collaboration of public health staff and leadership from 11 of the San Francisco Bay Area local health districts (LHDs) whose mission is to "transform public health practice for the purpose of eliminating health inequities using a broad spectrum of approaches that create healthy communities" (see: http://barhii.org/resources/sdoh-indicator-guide/introduction/). This BARHII indicator project began in February 2009 with the goal of developing indicators that demonstrate effects of SDOH and health inequities. They identified economic, social, physical, and service SDOH domains to focus on. For each domain, indicators and data sources are presented. For example, the service domain indicator is violent crime and the data source is Uniform Crime Reports. Income distribution falls within the economic domain and the data source used was the ACS.

Non-US data sources

The **World Values Survey (WVS)** (www.worldvaluessurvey.org/WVSContents.jsp) assesses political values, political orientation, and levels of political activity. Started in 1981 by a global network of social scientists wanting to know more about the impact of changing values on social and political life, this survey is a useful tool for identifying factors that influence health throughout the world. One of the key findings from the WVS is that what people believe has a primary influence on economic development, democracy, gender equality, and the extent to which societies have effective government (WVS, nd).

> Although economic factors often seem to play an important role in shaping cross cultural differences, it seems clear that they are not the only factors involved: these cultural differences seem to reflect the entire historical experience of given peoples, including political, social, technological, geographic, and other factors as well as economic influences.
>
> (Inglehart, Basañez, & Moreno, 1998, p. 5)

The **World Bank LAC Equity Lab** provides up-to-date data on poverty, inequality, and shared prosperity in the Latin America and the Caribbean (LAC) region (World Bank, nd). The equity lab includes indicators such as poverty, shared prosperity, income inequality, economic growth, labor markets, equality of opportunities, gender, and ethnicity.

The **Institute for Health Metrics and Evaluation** provides data visualizations using the SDOH for countries throughout the world (https://vizhub.healthdata.org/sdh/). Determinants include antenatal care visits, immunization coverage, education, and skilled birth attendance. Locations include global, high-income countries, and Latin American and Caribbean.

The **Canadian Index of Wellbeing (CIW)** is based on eight domains: community vitality, demographic engagement, education, environment, healthy populations, leisure and culture, living standards, and time use (https://uwaterloo.ca/canadian-index-wellbeing/what-we-do/domains-and-indicators). Indicators follow previous research and include 64 key social, health, economic, and environmental indicators that are known to promote overall quality of life in populations. Examples of indicators include percentage of populations that report a strong sense of belonging to community, percentage of women in Federal Parliament, average expenditure per public-school student, ground-level ozone, percentage of population that rates overall health as good or excellent, average percentage of time spent on previous day in arts and cultural activities, after tax median income, and percentage of population between the ages of 25 and 64 working over 50 hours per week at main job.

Primary data collection examples

If you plan on collecting primary data in your evaluation, below are some examples of how other public health programs have conceptualized this process.

The **Social Needs Screening Toolkit** combines guidelines from the IOM and Centers for Medicare and Medicaid Services (CMMS) to screen patient social needs. Essential domains include food insecurity, housing instability, utility needs, financial resource strain, transportation challenges, exposure to violence, and sociodemographic information (Health Leads, 2018). In primary care settings there are several SDOH tools that have been used to measure SDOH.

The IOM developed social and behavioral domains and measures for screening and follow-up, as shown in Table 4.2.

The CMMS developed the **Accountable Health Communities instrument (AHC)** (https://innovation.cms.gov/Files/worksheets/ahcm-screeningtool.pdf). This instrument includes five core domains: housing instability, food insecurity, transportation related problems, utility help needs, and interpersonal safety. Supplemental AHC domains are financial strain, employment, family and community support, education, physical activity, substance use, mental health, and disabilities.

The National Association of Community Health Centers developed a **Protocol for Responding to and Assessing Patient Assets, Risks and Experiences (PRAPARE)** (www.nachc.org/wp-content/uploads/2018/05/PRAPARE_One_Pager_Sept_2016.pdf). This assessment tool includes questions about family and home, money and resources, social and emotional health, and additional questions about incarceration, refugee status, safety, and violence.

Table 4.2 Social and behavioral domains and measures

Domain	Measure	Frequency
Race or Ethnic Group	Race, Hispanic, Latino, or Spanish origin	At intake
Education	Highest level school completed; highest degree earned	At intake
Financial Strain	Difficulty paying for food, housing, medical care, heat	At intake, follow-up
Stress	Feeling restless, nervous, anxious, unable to sleep	At intake, follow-up
Depression	Past two weeks little interests in pleasure, feeling down, depressed, hopeless	At intake, follow-up
Physical Activity	Days per week moderate exercise, minutes engaged	At intake, follow-up
Tobacco Use	Lifetime cigarette use, current cigarette/tobacco use	At intake, follow-up
Alcohol Use	Frequency of alcohol intake, daily intake, binge drinking	At intake, follow-up
Social Connections or Isolation	Frequency of talking and gathering with friends, attending church services, attending meetings or organizations	At intake, follow-up
Intimate Partner Violence	Past year humiliated or emotionally abused by partner/ex-partner, afraid, physically hurt	At intake, follow-up
Census-tract Median Income		

Source: Adapted from Adler & Stead (2015).

The **Center for Health Care Strategies Inc** developed a self-sufficiency outcomes matrix that assesses 12 SDOH areas, housing, employment, income, legal, mental health, substance abuse, health care coverage, stability, community involvement, parental supports, transportation, and health care. Response categories are based the lowest level of 1 or "in crisis" to the highest level of 5 or "empowered and thriving" (www.chcs.org/media/OneCare-Vermont-Self-Sufficiency-Outcome-Matrix_102517.pdf). Although this was developed for use in primary care settings, it could be used in a variety of community environments to identify resources and match individuals with resources available.

In other areas of SDOH data collection, researchers developed an 11-item scale to measure reflexive anti-racism at the University of Melbourne (Paradies, Franklin, & Kowal, 2013). This scale was developed for White anti-racists working with Australian Indigenous populations and communities. Constructs in the scale include racism, culture, structure, and agency items. Malecha and colleagues conducted a systematic review of material needs of emergency department patients (Malecha, Williams, Kunzler, et al., 2018).

They found patients have a high level of material needs—SDOH focused evaluations could help address these needs through appropriate screening and interventions. Just as with the screening tools listed above, the authors examined homelessness, poverty, housing insecurity, housing quality, food insecurity, unemployment, difficulty paying health care costs, and difficulty with basic expenses.

SDOH data in community settings

There are multiple SDOH focus areas in community settings. Marmot (2005) urges us to explore thriving populations using health status indicators as opposed to an economic well-being measure like the gross national product (GNP), average income, or consumption patterns. How healthy are people and what factors determine their health? Evidence suggests it is a mix of determinants, not just one. Think about the case of values as they influence social and political life and health. This mix of determinants has been documented in a variety of ways. Consider these indices below.

The **National Equity Atlas** indicators include demographics, economic vitality, readiness, and connectedness, and economic benefits of equity (https://nationalequityatlas.org/). The Diversity Index is available through the National Equity Atlas and measures neighborhood-level segregation, public-school segregation, income equality, and health equity. The National Equity Atlas includes hundreds of data points from public and private data sources for the 100 largest cities, the 150 largest metropolitan regions, all 50 states, and the United States, as well as demographic projections through 2050 (National Equity Atlas, 2019).

The **Social Vulnerability Index (SVI)** was developed by the Agency for Toxic Substances Disease Registry (ATSDR) and can help communities prepare for disasters and crisis. Factors like poverty, limited access to transportation, and crowded housing impact a community's ability to respond. ATSDR defines these in their SVI, which uses geospatial tools to map communities that may need the greatest support during a natural disaster or crisis. SVI scores range from 0, meaning the lowest vulnerability, to 1, the highest vulnerability (https://svi.cdc.gov/index.html).

The **Health Equity Index (HEI)** is based on 141 indicators from 50 different sources that are linked to health status. Indicators are grouped by 13 categories and 7 SDOH. Developed by the Connecticut Association of Directors of Health (CADH), the HEI can illuminate conditions that cause poorer health, encourage collaboration, and promote focus on upstream conditions like policy and prevention. The HEI is illustrated in Figure 4.7.

What all these tools have in common is that they are focused on SDOH categories and domains that could be used to assess changes in SDOH as a result of a public health intervention or program.

Now that we have a solid understanding of what SDOH data looks like and how to find it, let's move to how to analyze SDOH data for PHE.

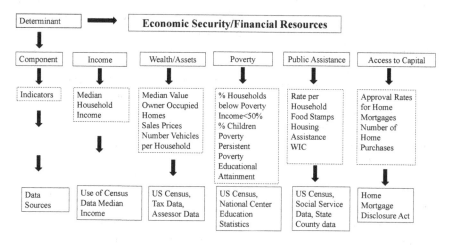

Figure 4.7 Health equity index and SDOH.

Source: Adapted from the Health Equity Index (Health Equity Alliance, 2010).

Analyzing data

Once you know the kinds of data that you will use in your evaluation, I recommend reviewing the data to make sure it is accurate and reflects the evaluation's needs and purpose. Analyzing and preparing data will depend on the kind of data that you have. If you are using primary data you will want to create a log for data, check for accuracy, create a database, enter the data into a computer, transform data, and then prepare to analyze it. It is always a good idea to create a data analysis plan (see Kelley, 2018, Appendix B) and create a plan for managing the data. Several resources are available for analyzing data and presenting data based on the type of data that you have and your evaluation need. We will not review these at length, but here are some terms that you should be familiar with. A **statistic** is a number that describes a sample characteristic. **Data** can be characteristics or numbers. A **population** is a complete set of actual or potential observations in an evaluation. A **parameter** is a number that describes a population characteristic; sometimes people refer to this as a sample statistic. A **sample** is a subset of the population that is intentionally selected. A **random sample** is a subset of a sample selected in a random effort so that everyone has an equal chance of being selected. A **variable** is a term used to describe a data point that is being collected in the evaluation and might include age, gender, or activity. There are different levels of measurement used in SDOH evaluations, and examples include nominal, ordinal, interval, or ratio variables. Nominal data uses a name such as "male." Ordinal data consists of ordered scales that represent values such as very satisfied or very dissatisfied. Interval data consists of numeric scales with an equal value between scale numbers—interval scales do not have an absolute zero (consider the case of outdoor temperature). Ratio variable data has an absolute zero and provides the numeric value between units. An example of a ratio variable is height and weight. **Descriptive data** may include the mean, median, mode, frequency distribution, standard deviation and variance analysis. **Inferential data** can be used in evaluation to make generalizations about a population from which the sample was taken. Descriptive data may include a mean and standard deviation, in which case "*M*" represents the **mean** or the average value of a sample or population and "*SD*" represents the **standard deviation** or the square root of the variance. **Variance** is the average of square differences between observations and their means. **Statistical significance** is used to determine if there are differences in an outcome due to chance. **Chi-square tests** are used to compare two groups of categorical data. **T-tests** are used to answer the question, "Is the difference between two samples different (significant) enough to say that something else could have caused the difference?" **Correlation analysis** is used to describe the linear relationship between two variables and its strength. The "*r*" value will always be between $+1$ and -1 where a -1.00 represents a perfect negative linear relationship, and $+1.00$ represents a perfect positive linear relationship. **Analysis of Variance (ANOVA)** can be helpful in determining if there is a statistically significant difference between three or more groups based on mean scores (Kelley, 2018).

You will likely have SDOH evaluation questions that include more than one variable. An example of a **univariate analysis** question might be: "What was the average income among program participants?" A **bivariate analysis** question is: "Is there a difference in income levels between individuals involved in the program and those who are not involved in the program?" A **multivariate analysis** question is: "Can income be predicted by age, involvement in the program, level of education, and urban location?" You can see that to answer these questions we would need multiple data sources. The analysis then would depend on the data used to answer these questions. A univariate data analysis result to the first question might be expressed as a number or a mean with a standard deviation. A bivariate data analysis result for the second question might include use of contingency tables and chi-square tests to explore differences in mean income levels between the two groups. Finally, a multivariate data analysis might include a factor analysis, regression, cluster or discriminant analysis, or other statistical techniques. The result of multivariate analysis could be expressed as a *R*-square value, correlation, beta weights, or equivalent *R*-square. If you would like more information on how to analyze variables from a SDOH evaluation, there is a range of statistical software and resources available. Microsoft Excel is a common software used to analyze data; Excel is used for data visualization and basic statistics. Statistical Package for Social Sciences (SPSS) is useful for more advanced statistical operations such as multivariate analyses and provides graphs and tables to help visualize data. R, SAS, and Minitab may also be used. Other programs exist and finding the right statistical software to analyze SDOH data will depend on the analyses required, the level of expertise that the user has, and the funds available to purchase software.

Qualitative data

Qualitative data represents anything that is not numeric. Examples of qualitative data include photos, interviews, drawings, journals, focus groups, transcripts from these, videos, and other visual non-numeric data. If you have qualitative data, I encourage you to create a data analysis plan and identify the paradigm from which you will be analyzing data. We reviewed different paradigms early in this text, and this is where paradigms and theories can be useful. For example, an **inductive analysis** approach allows you to identify concepts, themes, and models based on what is emerging in the data. In contrast, **grounded theory** utilizes data collected to create a theory about what is happening in a given community or context. Two frequent approaches to analyzing qualitative data are analytic methods and content analysis. **Analytic** methods include coding, sorting, and identifying themes, relationships, and conclusions about the data. In contrast, content analysis is more flexible and focuses on the content of data with less analysis. **Coding** is a process of identifying short items of text or phrases in your data that correspond to the evaluation question. **Categories** may be used to group coded segments. **Themes** build on categories and relate to the evaluation question (Kelley, 2018).

When you combine qualitative and quantitative data this is called a mixed-method approach. It is likely that you will have both types of data in your evaluation, therefore know these and use these.

International considerations

Although most of the challenges and solutions have focused on SDOH in the United States, there are unique considerations for developing countries. First, most SDOH studies are conducted in developed countries, like the United States. Most of the world's poorest countries are in Africa. The conditions, and therefore SDOH, in one country in Africa can be very different than those in the United States or other developed countries. For example, abject poverty, tribalism, lack of good governance, the abuse of power, corruption, nepotism, cultural traditions that are harmful, professional immigration, lack of technical skills, illiteracy, gender-related violence, armed conflict, and colonial legacy are factors that individually or collectively impact the health of African people and drive inequalities in health (Eshetu & Woldesenbet, 2011). While the approaches and SDOH vary across countries, there is agreement that more research is needed to explore SDOH in the poorest countries in the world while moving toward health equity for all.

Challenges and solutions

There are some common challenges to SDOH focused evaluations that go beyond the need for data. First, not everyone is aware of the SDOH and their importance in improving population health. Second, you will likely need to find data that tells you more about how the selected SDOH links to the program or intervention that you are evaluating. Third, it is possible that the funding focus may not allow for evaluating SDOH. Fourth, it may be difficult to find literature, existing evidence or a theoretical basis that supports the SDOH focus selected (Regidor, 2006). Fifth, the time allocated for the evaluation (e.g. six months, one year or even five years) to develop strategies and/or interventions that target SDOH focus areas and see results may not be enough. Finally, there is the issue of sustainability.

Lack of awareness

We must first understand the SDOH and then seek to achieve health equity. Previous authors report differences in the level of awareness about the SDOH among people, health care providers, and community organizations—understanding is the first step in building awareness about SDOH.

There is an ongoing debate about screening for SDOH that may be related to the lack of awareness that people have about the SDOH (Sokol, Austin, Chandler, et al., 2019). Some experts feel that screening is unethical if there are not resources in place to address unmet social needs while others feel that the absence of SDOH screening is unethical because it fails to identify individuals who are in need of additional support and care (Gottlieb, Fichtenberg, & Adler, 2016).

In Australia, local governments have led public health education initiatives to increase awareness and understanding about SDOH. The result of these efforts is that most local government staff know what the SDOH are and understand that policies are needed to address SDOH in policy and planning initiatives (Lawless, Lane, Lewis, et al., 2017). In healthcare settings, the need for increased awareness has been noted. Paul Isabelli wrote about this in a 2018 article, "Are you considering the other 50% of your patients' health?" (Isabelli, 2018). He urges providers to consider SDOH as a solution that will improve population health and reduce healthcare costs. In an article published by the Society of General Internal Medicine in 2019, researchers conducted a scoping review to explore how undergraduate medical education students learn about SDOH (Doobay-Persaud, Adler, Bartell, et al., 2019). They found limited tools, practices, or assessment methodologies in place that document how students learn about SDOH.

Collins and colleagues explored ideological barriers associated with health inequalities among active citizens (Collins, Abelson, & Eyles, 2007). They found that support for addressing health inequalities was associated with awareness of the SDOH, liberal values, and some sociodemographic characteristics. Collins and team identified barriers for addressing SDOH, including a lack of SDOH awareness, narrow understanding of the influences of social determinants on health, resistance to deprioritizing health care, and conservative values (Collins et al., 2007). A potential solution to the lack of awareness about SDOH is raising public awareness through message framing, narratives, and visual imagery.

Integrating data into electronic health records

Most of this chapter focuses on limited data, so by now you have a good understanding of where to find SDOH data. Gold and colleagues write about the difficulty of integrating SDOH data into electronic healthcare records (EHRs) (Gold, Bunce, Cowburn, et al., 2018). In their 2016 pilot study of HER-based SDOH data tools at three community health centers including 1,130 patients, the researchers reported barriers to collecting SDOH data. The primary barrier in utilizing EHR tools to collect SDOH data is that they create a distorted view of the patient and there is a lack of staff experience in SDOH (Adler & Stead, 2015). SDOH data and its consequences may be unmanageable, resulting in a lack of follow-up regarding social needs.

Lack of funding

Deficit-focused funding does not allow for exploring upstream factors that contribute to health inequalities. Chronic underfunding of public health in the United States has resulted in significant challenges in achieving health equity for all. The Centers for Disease Control and Prevention is the leading public health agency in the United States. Their 2019 budget was $7.3 billion—but one-third of their budget was obligated for supporting the opioid epidemic, and just 11% of their overall budget was dedicated for funding prevention and public health initiatives that would address SDOH (Trust for America's Health [TFAH], 2019). Critics are calling attention to the SDOH and the lack of funding that will promote better health outcomes: "Social determinants account for 80 percent of health outcomes, yet funding to address them lags. Governments, non-governmental organizations, and community members must work together." (TFAH, 2019, p. 9).

The need for evidence

One of the key challenges with SDOH focused evaluations is the need for evidence, but there is a lack of evidence on interventions that work. To begin, we must first ask, what type of evidence or literature is needed? Working in Indigenous communities, one of the kinds of evidence that is cited frequently is the "Grandmothers Test." This form of evidence is not based on western theories or public health models, but rather the intuitive knowledge of elders from a community. The concept is that elders and community members often know what is needed, what works, and what does not work. On the flip side of this, there are federal, state, and academic institutions that build evidence through program implementation and evaluation, utilizing sophisticated models, experimental designs, longitudinal studies, and predictive models. How we arrive at the kinds of evidence that we need in SDOH focused evaluation will largely depend on who the evaluation is for. A key challenge facing SDOH focused initiatives is the difficulty linking program or intervention outcomes to a social determinant, structural or systems change, and various other targets.

Tobacco control example of evidence-based policy and practice

Much of the public literature calls for evidence-based policy and practice—yet typically this call is about providing multiple lines of evidence from research, observations, and qualitative studies that create a theoretical basis for a program, policy, or intervention. One example of a United States policy that required multiple lines of evidence is government regulation of tobacco sales, marketing, and use. Beginning in 1906 with the Food and Drug Act, government regulations did not reference tobacco products but in 1914 the government advised that tobacco was used to cure, mitigate, and prevent disease (CDC, 2019). In 1963 the Food and Drug Administration (FDA) felt that tobacco was not harmful. Moving forward two years, lines of evidence were converging, and epidemiology, animal experiments, clinical observations and chemical analysis forced public health officials and medical authorities to acknowledge the link between cigarette use and cancer (CDC, 2019). Even with multiple lines of irrefutable evidence, it was not until the Comprehensive Smoking Education Act of 1984 that the government required rotating health warning labels and biennial reports to Congress on smoking and health, and required the cigarette industry to provide lists of ingredients in cigarettes. Public law 100–202 in 1987 banned smoking on domestic airline flights that were six hours or less. The Synar Amendment to the Alcohol, Drug Abuse, and Mental Health Administration (ADAMHA) Reorganization Act of 1992 required all states to adopt and enforce restrictions on tobacco sales to minors. Similarly, the Pro-Children Act of 1994 required federally funded children services to be smoke free. Finally, the Family Smoking Prevention and Tobacco Control Act of 2009 granted the FDA regulatory authority to oversee tobacco products.

Converging lines of evidence in the case of tobacco made a clear case for policy change or upstream approaches to address the epidemic, yet not all public health problems have such clear evidence (Proctor, 2012). A key criticism of public health literature, and therefore evaluation, is that programs and interventions are implemented in small settings with similar populations that lack real-world application (Glasgow & Emmons, 2007) and thus never address the causes of the causes. Researchers and policy makers are calling for connections between population-level interventions and programs and drivers of health inequities.

Theoretical basis

Another consideration in conducting SDOH focused evaluation is the lack of theoretical basis or evidence for using socioeconomic position and for what aspect of economic advantage or higher socioeconomic position it is that leads to improved health outcomes (Regidor, 2006). For example, is it education, culture, norms, resources, or power that leads to health, or a combination of these things? If an intervention increases socioeconomic position, will this guarantee health equality? What if it does not? There are no guarantees that a SDOH focused evaluation will result in evidence of an effect on income inequality and reduced health inequalities, but we can understand more about how theories can be used in SDOH focused evaluation.

"Diffusion of innovations" is an underlying theory that guides innovation over time with members of a social system. Uptake evidence is assessed on several factors at each stage of the policy-making process. Consider a policy idea, that is then supported by evidence, knowledge, research, ideas, politics, and economics. Public health may use the evidence to introduce, apply, and interpret various approaches to SDOH. Finally, capacity to implement policy change is often based on the individual, organization, and systems policy level (Bowen & Zwi, 2005).

Time needed

Most evaluations are time bound—well, most things in life are as well. SDOH evaluations take time, and time is not always on our side. Let's consider the Localities Embracing and Accepting Diversity (LEAD) pilot program designed to address race-based discrimination and improve the health of Aboriginal and migrant communities in Australia through social and economic participation (Ferdinand, Paradies, & Kehlaher, 2013). Previous work has linked self-reported discrimination to poorer health outcomes while social conditions that embrace cultural diversity promote better health outcomes (Paradies, 2006). This innovative program is based on a partnership model that involves mainstream organizations in the development of community-level interventions that target settings where racism occurs, educational settings, workplaces, sports, recreation, and retail settings. One of the key challenges reported by designers of LEAD is the time it takes to develop strategies within communities and partnerships that address race-based discrimination.

Sustainability

A primary challenge facing public health initiatives in general is the need for sustainability of efforts beyond implementation. Addressing sustainability early in program development is a must for SDOH focused programs. Routinization of programs within organizations may lead to better program-related organizational routines. Education about SDOH and addressing stigma and misperceptions about power and health may increase support for programming and future efforts.

Remember the LEAD project that we just read about? One of the LEAD project's primary concerns was the sustainability of the councils beyond the funding cycles. Partnerships with funding agencies and implementing programs or partners can help ensure a program's reach and sustainability through dissemination and knowledge sharing across networks, policy, and practices (Ferdinand et al., 2013).

Solutions

Use of a population health approach

With these challenges in mind, and there may be more ... Canada's Population Health Template measures SDOH and their interactions with health outcomes (www.phac-aspc.gc.ca/ph-sp/pdf/discussion-eng.pdf) and this is a potential solution. **Population health** simply means the health of a population based on multiple health status indicators. These indicators are influenced by multiple individual and community-level conditions. Canada's Population Health Template includes eight key elements and actions that define a population health approach (Health Canada, 2001).

1   Focus on the health of populations
2   Address SDOH and their interactions
3   Base decisions on evidence
4   Increase upstream investments
5   Apply multiple strategies
6   Collaborate across sectors and levels
7   Employ mechanisms for public involvement in strategies and purpose
8   Demonstrate accountability for health outcomes

If we apply these elements to SDOH focused evaluations, we can clearly see how multiple strategies are needed to promote health equity. How do we operationalize these elements in SDOH focused evaluations? Let's take a closer look.

How do evaluators focus on the health of populations? First, determine what indicators can be used to measure health status, then measure and analyze health status and health inequities to identify health issues and targets for SDOH programming and interventions. Know the context, conditions, trends, and characteristics of a population.

How do evaluators address determinants of health and interactions between health and conditions? First determine which indicators will be used to measure determinants, then measure and analyze determinants and explore their interactions, then link these to health determinants.

How can evaluators use evidence to formulate plans and decision making? First, use the best available evidence at all times. Have criteria that outline why some evidence will be included while other evidence will be excluded. Use multiple data sources and mixed evaluation methods (both qualitative and quantitative data). Know what interventions might be effective and assess their effectiveness in the program. Share results with policy makers, the scientific community, and others to ensure updates of findings to influence policy change.

How can evaluators support upstream investments? The first step is understanding what upstream investments look like and the time needed to change stream conditions. Evaluators can influence other programs, policies, and sectors by drawing on the evidence and demonstrating SDOH and structural inequalities that need to change.

Why is it important to use multiple strategies in a SDOH focused evaluation? There are multiple factors that contribute to health inequity. Use of multiple strategies can help build an evidence base for SDOH interventions while providing insight into the interactions between socioeconomic, structural, cultural, behavioral, environmental, and physiological conditions that create poor health outcomes.

How do evaluators collaborate with other partners and programs? Partnerships are at the core of evaluation, and participatory evaluation methods are necessary to understand conditions and design effective evaluation strategies. Partnerships and collaborations create support, visibility, leadership, and accountability that are needed for SDOH evaluations.

Why is it important to involve the public? Community involvement is necessary because it is one way that evaluators can learn about conditions, promote equity and shared decision making, and understand what the community's interests and needs are for SDOH programming and evaluation. Community involvement also increases health literacy and awareness about SDOH.

Who is accountable for health outcomes and what is the role of the evaluator in this? Everyone is accountable for health outcomes. Having access to health is a fundamental right and an issue of social justice that does not sit on the shoulders of just one person or a handful of people. Health Canada (2001) recommends developing a result-based accountability framework that is agreed upon by the evaluator and all program partners. This framework includes a clear statement of roles and responsibilities, resources, performance strategies, schedule of evaluation, and reporting provisions that promote transparency and accountability. From the start, document baseline measures and targets for health improvements. Make evaluation part of each program within an organization or institution. Health Impact Assessment tools (see Appendix C) can help document changes in health outcomes over time. Finally, promote accountability by disseminating the results of SDOH evaluations. Results demonstrate impacts and document areas of need for future work. Examples of reporting results include population health reports, case studies, and best practices that promote a population health approach.

Ten essential public health services

The 10 essential public health services are another potential solution for SDOH focused evaluations. These are driven by the Centers for Disease Control and Prevention and are focused on clarifying and supporting the roles of public health agencies as they address structural inequalities and SDOH. CDC defines public health systems as the following:

- Public health agencies at state and local levels
- Healthcare providers
- Public safety agencies
- Human service and charity organizations

- Education and youth development organizations
- Recreation and arts-related organizations
- Economic and philanthropic organizations
- Environmental agencies and organizations (CDC, 2019)

To begin, these services are based on a cyclical process of assessment, policy development, and assurance. Below is a list of each service recommended:

1 Monitor health status to identify and solve community health problems.
2 Diagnose and investigate health problems and health hazards in the community.
3 Inform, educate, and empower people about health issues.
4 Mobilize community partnerships and action to identify and solve health problems.
5 Develop policies and plans that support individual and community health efforts.
6 Enforce laws and regulations that protect health and ensure safety.
7 Link people to needed personal health services and assure the provision of health care when otherwise unavailable.
8 Assure a competent public and personal health care workforce.
9 Evaluate effectiveness, accessibility, and quality of personal and population-based health services.
10 Use research for new insights and innovative solutions to health problems (CDC, 2019).

Evaluators may be familiar with these services and guidance, but how do they relate to SDOH focused evaluations?

- First, monitor health status to identify and solve community health problems. Evaluators can do this by including SDOH measures (mentioned throughout this text) to address poor health outcomes and inequities in health. Community Health Assessments are one tool that measure SDOH via community partners involved in public health efforts.
- Second, diagnose and investigate health problems and health hazards in the community. Evaluators can support this by encouraging the use of community-level interventions that inform policy and practice.
- Third, inform, educate, and empower people about health issues. Evaluators play an important role as educators about the SDOH. Use of culturally and linguistically appropriate approaches can help address SDOH and acknowledge structural racism, discrimination, and stigma that impact health equity.
- Fourth, mobilize community partnerships and action to identify and solve health problems. Evaluators can do this by working with multiple partners who have a vested interest or knowledge base about the SDOH being evaluated.
- Fifth, develop policies and plans that support individual and community health efforts. Evaluators collect and report on evidence that can be used in

the uptake of SDOH policies that support health equity. Evaluators may leverage partnerships and identify policies from other disciplines to support SDOH approaches.

- Sixth, enforce laws and regulations that protect health and ensure safety. Evaluators can support communities and organizations as they enforce laws and regulations that support health equity and healthy conditions. Zoning laws are just one of the many examples where evaluations have directed improvements to neighborhood conditions to support health and safety (consider access to physical space, lighting, and abandoned buildings/codes).
- Seventh, link people to needed personal health services and assure the provision of health care when otherwise unavailable. Evaluators with knowledge of health program services can direct and support programs as they address individual health and population health needs—for example, social services programs, and Medicaid benefits.
- Eighth, assure a competent public and personal health care workforce. Evaluators can do this by encouraging training in the SDOH and hiring workers who reflect the target population of interest. For example, if an evaluator is working with a Latino community, it would be helpful if they were Latino and from that community. If this is not possible, then the evaluator would need to have knowledge about the community, their language, culture, norms, and needs.
- Ninth, evaluate effectiveness, accessibility, and quality of personal and population-based health services. Evaluators help demonstrate effectiveness by selecting appropriate evaluation designs, based on the resources, time, and expertise available. Evaluators generate reports, information, and recommendations for quality improvement that may address underlying causes of poor health outcomes.
- Tenth, use research for new insights and innovative solutions to health problems. Evaluators can advocate for research agendas and funding that supports a SDOH approach. Use of participatory and empowerment evaluation methods, and of evidence-based practices, is also recommended (CDC, 2019).

In sum, evaluators play an important role in ensuring that public health programs and services address SDOH and health inequities. These steps and recommendations provide insight into how a population health approach drives SDOH solutions and advocacy.

Summary

Michael Marmot asks one question at the beginning of this chapter, "Why is the life expectancy 48 years longer in Japan than in Sierra Leone or 20 years shorter in Australian Aboriginal and Torres Strait Islander peoples than in other Australians?" While this chapter did not answer Marmot's question completely, we do know there are unique challenges and strengths associated with each community throughout the world. We know that inequalities in health are a symptom of a much larger problem about power and resources. SDOH focused evaluations are a first step in restoring power, giving voice and opportunity to those who have been ignored, and creating upstream public health programs that close the life expectancy gap.

This chapter began with an overview of challenges that evaluators may experience as they utilize SDOH focused evaluations. These challenges include limited data, difficulty linking programs to results, limited evidence-based evaluations that utilize a SDOH approach, and difficulty comparing or measuring SDOH factors between countries and among populations. This chapter also outlined solutions for SDOH focused evaluation and screening tools that can help identify SDOH.

Points to remember

1   Lack of awareness and understanding may lead to challenges in SDOH focused evaluation.
2   Increasing SDOH awareness within individuals, organizations, communities, health care providers, and nations is needed.
3   There are multiple ways to conceptualize SDOH focused evaluations, and utilizing multiple data sets, approaches, and paradigms will help. The HEI provides one of the many examples of how to connect determinants, indicators, and data sources.
4   Data is both a challenge and a strength of SDOH focused evaluations. Knowing how to access SDOH data and the interplay of SDOH and outcomes of interest is an important skill set for evaluators.

Additional reading and resources

Agency for Toxic Substance Disease Registry Vulnerability Index
https://svi.cdc.gov/index.html

American Community Survey US Data
www.census.gov/programs-surveys/acs/

Bureau of Justice Statistics
https://bjs.gov/

Centers for Disease Control Health Equity Workbook
www.cdc.gov/nccdphp/dch/programs/healthycommunitiesprogram/tools/pdf/
SDOH-workbook.pdf

Federal Bureau of Investigation Crime Related Data US
www.fbi.gov/

Health Begins Upstream Communication Toolkit
www.healthbegins.org/resources-for-social-determinants-of-health.html

Health Resources Services Administration
https://data.hrsa.gov/topics/health-workforce/shortage-areas

Social Interventions Research Evaluation Network SDOH Screening Tools
https://sirenetwork.ucsf.edu/tools-resources/screening-tools

Ten Essential Public Health Services
www.cdc.gov/publichealthgateway/publichealthservices/essentialhealthservices.html

Chapter questions

1 List three challenges of SDOH focused evaluations.
2 Describe two different types of data and how they could be used in SDOH evaluation efforts.
3 List two SDOH screening tools. In what settings would these tools be used? Describe the strengths and weaknesses of each tool.
4 What are potential challenges of utilizing multiple data sets to identify SDOH in public health evaluation?

Activities on the web

1 Go to the American Community Survey US Data (www.census.gov/programs-surveys/acs/). Identify one data set available from the ACS that could be used in a SDOH focused evaluation that has not been discussed in this chapter. Describe your rationale for selecting this data set and the strengths and limitations of the data as they relate to the SDOH.
2 Search the web for agencies, organizations, or associations that are funding SDOH programming. Identify three additional resources from this search that could potentially be used to support SDOH efforts.
3 Go to the Bureau of Justice Statistics website (https://bjs.gov/). Review arrests and crime data for racial groups in the United States. Discuss disparities in arrest rates based on percentage of the populations and describe potential SDOH programs that could address discriminatory criminal justice programs and staff.
4 Go to the IHME website data visualizations (https://vizhub.healthdata.org/sdh/) and review indicators based on determinants, outcomes, sex, and region. How might these visualizations be used in a SDOH evaluation?

References

Adler, N. E., & Stead, W. W. (2015). Patients in context: EHR capture of social and behavioral determinants of health. *New England Journal of Medicine, 372*(8), 698–701.

Agency for Toxic Substance Disease Registry. (2015). *Evaluation methods: Community engagement.* Retrieved from: www.atsdr.cdc.gov/communityengagement/pce_program_methods.html.

American Community Survey. (2017). Selected housing characteristics. ACS 5-year estimates data profiles. Retrieved from: https://data.census.gov/cedsci/table?q=&d=ACS% 205-Year%20Estimates%20Data%20Profiles&table=DP04&tid=ACSDP5Y2017.DP0 4&y=2017&hidePreview=true&g=&lastDisplayedRow=159.

American Community Survey. (2019). 2013–2017 community facts, New Mexico. Housing characteristics, education, income. Retrieved from: https://factfinder.census. gov/faces/nav/jsf/pages/index.xhtml.

American Housing Survey. (2019). 2017 national income characteristics, education of householder. Retrieved from: www.census.gov/programs-surveys/ahs/data/interactive/ ahstablecreator.html?s_areas=00000&s_year=2017&s_tablename=TABLE9&s_ bygroup1=20&s_bygroup2=14&s_filtergroup1=3&s_filtergroup2=1.

Bowen, S., & Zwi, A. B. (2005). Pathways to "evidence-informed" policy and practice: A framework for action. *PLoS Medicine, 2*(7), e166. doi:10.1371/journal.pmed.0020166.

Bureau of Justice Statistics. (2019). Prisoners in 2017: Imprisonment rates. NCJ252156. Retrieved from: www.bjs.gov/content/pub/pdf/p17_sum.pdf.

Bureau of Labor Statistics. (2018). Expanded state employment status demographic data. Retrieved from: www.bls.gov/lau/ex14tables.htm.

Center for American Women and Politics. (2019). Women in elective office 2019. Facts. Retrieved from: www.cawp.rutgers.edu/women-elective-office-2019.

Centers for Disease Control and Prevention. (2019). *The ten essential public health services.* Retrieved from: www.cdc.gov/publichealthgateway/publichealthservices/ essentialhealthservices.html.

Chappelow, J. (2019). Gini Index. What is the Gini Index? *Economy Investopedia.* Retrieved from: www.investopedia.com/terms/g/gini-index.asp.

Collins, P. A., Abelson, J., & Eyles, J. D. (2007). Knowledge into action? Understanding ideological barriers to addressing health inequalities at the local level. *Health Policy, 80*(1), 158–171.

Doobay-Persaud, A., Adler, M., Bartell, T., Sheneman, N., Martinez, M., Mangold, K., ... & Sheehan, K. (2019). Teaching the social determinants of health in undergraduate medical education: A scoping review. *Journal of General Internal Medicine, 34*(5), 720–730. doi:10.1007/s11606-019-04876-0.

Environmental Protection Agency. (2019). Air quality statistics by city, 2018. Ozone 8-hour average parts per million. Retrieved from: www.epa.gov/ground-level-ozone-pollution.

Eshetu, E. B., & Woldesenbet, S. A. (2011). Are there particular social determinants of health for the world's poorest countries? *African Health Sciences, 11*(1), 108–115.

Federal Bureau of Investigations. (2018). *Crime in the United States.* Available from: https://ucr.fbi.gov/crime-in-the-u.s/2018/crime-in-the-u.s.-2018.

Ferdinand, A. S., Paradies, Y., & Kelaher, M. A. (2013). The role of effective partnerships in an Australian place-based intervention to reduce race-based discrimination. *Public Health Reports, 128*(6, Suppl. 3), 54–60.

Glasgow, R. E., & Emmons, K. M. (2007). How can we increase translation of research into practice? Types of evidence needed. *Annual Review of Public Health, 28*, 413–433.

Gold, R., Bunce, A., Cowburn, S., Dambrun, K., Dearing, M., Middendorf, M., ... & Davis, J. (2018). Adoption of social determinants of health EHR tools by community health centers. *The Annals of Family Medicine, 16*(5), 399–407.

Gottlieb, L., Fichtenberg C., & Adler N. (2016). Screening for social determinants of health. *JAMA, 316*(23), 2552.

Hajat, A., Hsia, C., & O'Neill, M. S. (2015). Socioeconomic disparities and air pollution exposure: A global review. *Current Environmental Health Reports*, *2*(4), 440–450. doi:10.1007/s40572-015-0069-5.

Health Canada. (2001). The Population Health Template. Retrieved from: www.phac-aspc. gc.ca/ph-sp/pdf/discussion-eng.pdf.

Health Equity Alliance (2010). *About the Health Equity Index*. Available from: www. sdoh.org/about/hei.

Health Leads. (2018). Social Needs Screening Toolkit. Retrieved from: https://healthleadsusa. org/resources/the-health-leads-screening-toolkit/?tfa_next=%2Fresponses%2Flast_succe ss%26sid%3Dc62351e4c7bf609d210d0cb79d4da686.

Health Resources and Services Administration. (2019). Health professional shortage areas by type and discipline. Retrieved from: https://data.hrsa.gov/topics/health-work- force/shortage-areas.

Hillemeier, M., Lynch, J., Harper, S., & Casper, M. (2004). Data set directory of social determinants of health at the local level. Atlanta, GA: US Department of Health and Human Services, Centers for Disease Control and Prevention. Retrieved from: www. cdc.gov/dhdsp/docs/data_set_directory.pdf.

Inglehart, R. F., Basañez, M., & Moreno, A. (1998). *Human values and beliefs: A cross-cultural sourcebook*. Retrieved from https://ebookcentral.proquest.com.

Isabelli, P. (2018). Are you considering the other 50% of your patient's health? *Health Management Technology*, (July–August), p. 18. Retrieved from: https://link.gale.com/ apps/doc/A547630581/CDB?u=gree35277&sid=CDB&xid=4636f402.

Kelley, A. (2018). Evaluation in rural communities. London, UK: Routledge. doi:10.4324/9780429458224.

Krieger, N., Chen, J. T., Waterman, P. D., Soobader, M. J., Subramanian, S. V., & Carson, R. (2002). Geocoding and monitoring of US socioeconomic inequalities in mortality and cancer incidence: Does the choice of area-based measure and geographic level matter? The Public Health Disparities Geocoding Project. *American Journal of Epidemiology*, *156*(5), 471–482. doi:10.1093/aje/kwf068.

Lawless, A., Lane, A., Lewis, F. A., Baum, F., & Harris, P. (2017). Social determi- nants of health and local government: Understanding and uptake of ideas in two Australian states. *Australian and New Zealand Journal of Public Health*, *41*(2), 204–209.

Lofters, A. K., Schuler, A., Slater, M., Baxter, N. N., Persaud, N., Pinto, A. D., ... & Kiran, T. (2017). Using self-reported data on the social determinants of health in primary care to identify cancer screening disparities: Opportunities and challenges. *BMC Family Practice*, *18*(1), 31.

Lofters, A. K., Shankardass, K., Kirst, M., & Quiñonez, C. (2011). Sociodemographic data collection in healthcare settings: An examination of public opinions. *Medical Care*, *49*(2), 193–199.

Malecha, P., Williams, J., Kunzler, N., Goldfrank, L., Alter, H., & Doran, K. (2018). Material needs of emergency department patients: A systematic review. *Academic Emergency Medicine*, *25*(3), 330–359. doi:10.1111/acem.13370.

Marmot, M. (2005). Social determinants of health inequalities. *The Lancet*, 365(9464), 1099–1104.

National Center for Education Statistics (2019). State revenue per pupil by source. 2015–2016. Retrieved from: https://nces.ed.gov/ccd/elsi/expressTables.aspx.

National Equity Atlas (2019). Indicators. United States. Retrieved from: https://national equityatlas.org/indicators/Racial_generation_gap.

Paradies, Y. (2006). A systematic review of empirical research on self-reported racism and health. *International Journal of Epidemiology*, *35*(4), 888–901.

Paradies, Y., Franklin, H., & Kowal, E. (2013). Development of the reflexive antiracism scale–Indigenous. *Equality, Diversity and Inclusion: An International Journal*, *32*(4), 348–373.

Proctor, R. (2012). The history of the discovery of the cigarette–lung cancer link: Evidentiary traditions, corporate denial, global toll. *Tobacco Control*, *21*(2), 87–91.

Regidor, E. (2006). Social determinants of health: A veil that hides socioeconomic position and its relationship with health. *Journal of Epidemiology and Community Health*, *60*(10), 896–901. Retrieved from www.jstor.org/stable/40665472. doi:10.1136/¡ ech.2005.044859.

Sokol, R., Austin, A., Chandler, C., Byrum, E., Bousquette, J., Lancaster, C., ... & Brevard, K. (2019). Screening children for social determinants of health: A systematic review. *Pediatrics*, *144*(4), e20191622. doi:10.1542/peds.2019–1622.

Trust for America's Health. (2019). *The impact of chronic underfunding on America's public health system: Trends, risks, and recommendations.* Available from: www.tfah. org/wp-content/uploads/2019/04/TFAH-2019-PublicHealthFunding-06.pdf.

US Agency for International Development (2010). *Performance monitoring and evaluation tips for selecting performance indicators.* Retrieved from: https://pdf.usaid.gov/ pdf_docs/pnadw106.pdf.

US Bureau of the Census. (2019). Current population survey, annual social and economic supplements. Retrieved from: www.census.gov/data/tables/time-series/demo/income-poverty/historical-income-inequality.html.

US Census Bureau (2019). 2017 State and local government finance historical datasets and tables. Retrieved from: www.census.gov/data/datasets/2017/econ/local/public-use-datasets.html.

World Bank (nd). LAC Equity Lab: Income inequality–income distribution. Retrieved from: www.worldbank.org/en/topic/poverty/lac-equity-lab1/income-inequality/income-distribution.

World Values Survey (nd). Findings and insights. Retrieved from: www.worldvalues survey.org/WVSContents.jsp.

5 SDOH program examples

Learning objectives

After reading this chapter, you should be able to:

- List solid SDOH facts that inform public health programming
- Describe policies and programs with a scientific evidence base that can improve health
- Explain what Health in All Policies means and its importance to SDOH focused programming
- Differentiate between racism and discrimination and the role of each in SDOH program efforts
- Discuss implicit bias and how this relates to SDOH
- List SDOH programming examples in the private sector and their impact on health

Up until this point, we have been reading about evaluation, SDOH history, theories, paradigms, frameworks, challenges, solutions, screening tools, and overall approaches. It is now time to explore how programs are addressing SDOH in the real world. I hope by now you have come to understand that the SDOH are significant and that programs that target SDOH have the potential to reduce health inequalities and promote justice.

> No causes are themselves uncaused, however, which means that when we think about what causes lung cancer or even smoking, we should think not just in terms of how individuals "decide" to start smoking, but rather in terms of larger, more web like threads of causation. We have to look at the cigarette epidemic—and therefore lung cancer—as facilitated by long causal chains of a sociopolitical, technical, molecular and agricultural nature. If cigarettes cause cancer, then so do the machines that roll cigarettes and the companies that supply the "filters", "flavorings" and paper. We need to better understand such webs or networks if we are to be more creative in finding ways to reduce the toll from this, the world's deadliest malignancy.
>
> (Proctor, 2012, p. 91)

Solid facts

With so many causes and causes of causes, it might feel overwhelming to select just one. Understanding causation and associations between SDOH and poorer health outcomes is an important first step. In Chapter 1 we reviewed the SDOH and significant events in world history that led to where we are at today—the need for SDOH focused evaluation. We introduced the 10 solid SDOH facts from Richard Wilkinson and Michael Marmot's work (2003). These solid facts give insight into the kinds of public health programming needed to address health inequalities. Let's explore these in greater detail.

1 Social gradient—Poor social and economic conditions affect health, leading to shorter life expectancy.
2 Stress—Social and psychological conditions may cause long-term stress that leads to anxiety, insecurity, social isolation, lack of control. Stress hormones and the nervous system trigger fight or flight responses and, over time, affect the cardiovascular and immune system response, leading to infections, diabetes, high blood pressure, stroke, depression, and aggression.
3 Early life—Beginning during pregnancy, maternal stress, nutrition, substance use, exercise, and care impact fetal development and health. Infant exposure and development continue throughout early life.
4 Social exclusion—Absolute poverty, relative poverty, and social exclusion translate to poor quality of life and shorter lifespans.
5 Work—Stress in the workplace impacts health. Limited opportunities to use skills and limited decision making impact health by way of increased lower back pain, sickness, and cardiovascular disease.
6 Unemployment—Places people at risk for premature death, impacts mental health, and increases risk factors for heart disease.
7 Social support—Lack of support places people at risk for premature death and poorer chances of surviving a heart attack.
8 Addiction—Linked with social and economic disadvantage, associated with accidents, violence, poisoning, injury, and suicide.
9 Food—High fat intake, excess intake, food poverty, and access impact health.
10 Transport—Limited use of cycling, walking, and public transportation may take away from health because of increased accidents, decreased social contact, and increases in air pollution.

With these facts in mind, in this chapter we will explore examples of how public health programs are building health equity and health equality using SDOH. In Chapter 3 we presented SDOH program goals from the Kaiser Foundation, and these SDOH goals are evident in various SDOH programs that we will review. They include community cohesion, access to health care and prevention, food access and nutrition, economic opportunities, education and childhood development, housing, built environment, transportation, and environmental justice.

Evaluation can help us determine if goals have been met while building an evidence base for SDOH.

Chapter 4 discussed the lack of evidence for SDOH programming as a challenge. One of the major challenges that evaluators experience is determining what actions are needed to build justice, equality, well-being, and population health and then weaving these into a program evaluation plan.

Programs with scientifically supported evidence

The Robert Wood Johnson Foundation (RWJF) summarizes 161 policies and programs that can improve health with scientifically supported evidence (RWJF, 2019b). Criteria used to determine if a policy or program is scientifically supported are as follows: one or more systematic reviews, three experimental studies, and three quasi-experimental studies with matched concurrent comparisons. Other characteristics include strong designs and statistically significant findings that are favorable toward the health or policy outcome of interest. Briefly, a **systematic review** summarizes results of carefully designed studies like controlled trials and provides quality evidence and recommendations for health. **Experimental studies** are characterized by random assignment of participants to one of two or more groups. Evaluators then explore differences in outcomes that can be linked to an intervention based on group assignment. One example of an experimental study is a randomized control trial. **Quasi-experimental** studies are nonrandomized interventions that seek to show causality between an intervention and an outcome (Harris, McGregor, Perencevich, et al., 2006). **Statistical significance** is used to determine if there are differences in an outcome due to chance. Most often significance levels are set at (p) 0.95. This means that there is a 95% chance that the results are true, or $1-p$. Significance is reported using (p) 0.001 or 0.05; these numbers mean there is a 0.001% or 5% chance the results are not true (Kelley, 2018; Rice, 1989). Different statistical tests will report p values for you to consider.

While not all the RWJF policies and programs are upstream approaches, some of them are. Let's explore some of the programs and policies with an upstream focus that are scientifically supported, and have a direct impact on reducing disparities, as illustrated in Table 5.1.

With these evidence-based programs in mind, let's look at evidence-based policy as a program and institutional approach to building health equity.

Health in All Policies

Health in All Policies (HiAP) is an orientation to building health equity that is based on a principle that health is influenced by lifestyles and environments. HiAP supports the concept that health is linked to social, cultural, and environmental determinants that influence health. Thus, Health in All Policies is related to the different aspects of social and environmental factors that influence health.

Table 5.1 SDOH focus areas and scientifically supported program examples

SDOH Focus Area	Program Examples
Addiction	Mentoring programs, drug courts, internet-based tobacco cessation, mass media campaigns against alcohol impaired driving, tobacco use, syringe exchange, tobacco quit lines
Financial	Conditional cash transfer programs Latin America, supplemental social security, child care subsidies, financial assistance for working parents to pay for childcare, child support pass through, transitional jobs, workforce training, job corps, vocational training
Crime	Focused deterrence strategies, drug courts, mentoring to address delinquency, multi-systemic therapy, neighborhood watch, restorative justice
Education	College access programs, dropout prevention, dropout prevention teen moms, earned income tax credit, health career recruitment minority students, Incredible Years, mentoring high school graduation, charter school, physically active classrooms, summer learning
Early Childhood	Healthy Families America, home visiting programs, head start, full day kindergarten, preschool education
Environment	Streetscape design initiatives, soil conservation, flexible work scheduling, healthy home environment assessments, housing rehabilitation loan and grant programs, lead paint abatement, outdoor experiential education and wilderness therapy, public transportation, safe routes to school, swimming pool fencing
Food Access and Nutrition	Fruit and vegetable incentive programs, school breakfast, school gardens
Healthcare	Federally Qualified Health Centers, community health workers, culturally tailored educational programs, care coordination of systems, nurse–family partnership program, tobacco cessation, long term care elders, patient navigators, patient shared decision making, rural training medical education, school health programs, telemedicine
License, Zoning, Laws, Policies, Regulations	Raise price of tobacco, support flavor bans, protect indoor clean air, limited number and concentration of alcohol outlets by area, increase taxes, blood alcohol concentration laws, breath test check points, care seat enforcement, community policing, firearm licensing, hot spot policing, mental health benefits legislation, minimum drinking age laws, paid family leave, seatbelt laws, zoning regulations for land use
Parenting/ Families	Group based parenting programs, function family therapy, kinship foster care, family support for preschoolers
Social and Relational	Extracurricular activities, bullying prevention, positive behavioral interventions, school-based social and emotional instruction
Technology	Screen time interventions, text message health-based interventions

Source: RWJF, 2019.

Below are several examples of HiAP approaches that we can learn from as we consider SDOH programming.

The **Safe Routes to School National Partnership** integrated HiAP into the *Safe Routes to School Local Policy Guide* (Cowan, Hubsmith, & Ping, 2011) by incorporating health, physical activity, and safety into the Policy Guide. Using this approach allowed policymakers to be leaders in building healthy communities (Chriqui, Taber, Slater, et al., 2012). When people feel empowered and that they are contributing, this leads to improved health outcomes. This HiAP approach targets SDOH intervention points of work and transportation.

In 2006 Finland adopted the HiAP orientation to explore how health determinants are controlled by policies opposed to health outcomes. The **Finnish Initiative** builds on SDOH historical events like the Alma Ata Declaration that we learned about in Chapter 1. Beginning in 1970, Finland started taking action to improve diets in order to reduce morbidity and mortality associated with cardiovascular disease. Their goal was to influence policy making at all levels in Europe, national, regional and local (Puska, 2006). Results from HiAP efforts have led to legislation and major improvements in population health in the last 20 years; however, additional efforts are needed to close the health gap as health inequalities remain across social groups throughout Finland (Melkas, 2013). This HiAP approach targets SDOH intervention points of social gradients.

Universal access to medical care is a SDOH that is influenced by policy and benefits from an HiAP orientation. The American Academy of Family Physicians (AAFP) supports the statement that health is a basic human right for every person and that the right to health includes universal access to timely, acceptable, and affordable health care of appropriate quality (AAFP, 2018). In the last 20 years in the United States, several policies have been implemented to promote health as a basic human right, including the Children's Health Insurance Program (CHIP) and the Patient Protection and Affordable Care Act (ACA). Policies have extended access to health coverage for millions of Americans who were either uninsured, underinsured, or non-Medicare eligible (AAFP, 2018). Policy implications from the ACA are still being explored. One example from the ACA is with the state of Oregon. Oregon health care is delivered using 15 coordinated care organizations with a shared goal of improving population health and health outcomes and lowering costs. To meet this goal, Oregon developed seven quality improvement focus areas: improve behavioral health and physical coordination, improve prenatal and maternity care, reduce preventable hospitalizations, ensure appropriate care/settings, reduce costs by super users, address discrete health issues, and improve primary care for all populations. Oregon utilizes a multitiered strategy to address individual, community and policy level efforts that impact health (IOM, 2014). Universal medical care indirectly addresses all SDOH intervention points.

The **American Indian Cancer Foundation** HiAP is evident in the sacred traditional tobacco for healthy Native communities initiative. Melanie Plucinski, Policy Programs Manager at the Band River Band of Lake Superior Chippewa, presented work from the Tribal Health Equity Project. This project is working toward health equity through critical conversations with American Indians in Minnesota. Using a HiAP orientation, the American Indian Cancer Foundation is elevating equity through improved access to economic, educational, and political opportunities, capacity to make decisions that impact change, social and environmental safety, and culturally competent health care across all sectors (Plucinski, 2016). The Tribal Health Equity Project addresses social gradient, addiction, social support, and stress SDOH intervention points.

The **Centers for Disease Control and Prevention Health Impact in 5 Years (HI-5)** community initiative is a non-clinical, community-based approach that is addressing the SDOH by changing the context (www.cdc.gov/policy/hst/hi5/index.html). SDOH focus areas include early childhood education, clean diesel bus fleets, public transport systems, home improvement loans and grants, earned income tax credits, and water fluoridation (CDC, 2019). Through these efforts, CDC hopes that HI-5 will change the context for school-based programs to increase physical activity, promote violence prevention, promote safe routes to school, reduce motorcycle injures, increase tobacco control interventions, increase access to clean syringes, integrate pricing strategies for alcohol products, and implement multicomponent worksite obesity prevention programs. The HI-5 project addresses multiple SDOH intervention points.

Spotlight on programs that address SDOH

There are multiple programs addressing the SDOH. This section highlights some of these and provides insight into how evaluations target SDOH intervention points for population health and health equity.

Project DULCE (Developmental Understanding for Legal Collaboration for Everyone) was a pilot project designed to improve care of new-borns and their families with Boston Medical Center's Pediatrics Department. Focusing on upstream factors such as low income, high debts to assets ratio, and negative financial events, DULCE was developed using the Strengthening Families Protective Factors Framework and parts of the Medical–Legal partnerships approach. DULCE recruited families into intervention or control groups. Eligible families had babies from 0 to 6 months of age from 2010–2012. More than 90% were Latino or other underrepresented populations. Family specialists worked with the families to provide knowledge and training on child development milestones and problem solving. DULCE has now expanded into state and child welfare efforts, improvements in Medi-Cal enrollment for babies, and equitable immigration systems that promote family well-being (https://cssp.org/our-work/project/dulce#dulce-in-action).

Results from DULCE show a significant impact in the form of reduced emergency room visits. DULCE targets SDOH intervention points of early childhood development, health care access, and systems change.

Public Health–Seattle and King County (PHSKC) is building policies based on the science of early childhood development. Efforts at PHSKC were informed by the report published by the IOM and the National Research Council in 2000, *From Neurons to Neighbourhoods: The Science of Early Childhood Development* (IOM and National Research Council, 2000). PHSKC developed an intervention to improve the social and economic factors that strengthen early childhood development through public and private policies throughout the lifespan. Through innovative partnerships with state, local, and federal agencies, PHSKC identified five areas of focus for improving policy: nurturing relationships, family resources, childcare, neighborhood, and access to early interventions. Developing a policy agenda took one and a half years and was a difficult process. Leaders of the PHSKC described how it was difficult to focus on social and economic contextual factors and on how to make incremental steps toward structural changes in the environment (housing, adequate food, health care, childcare, and financial resources). While the goal of PHSKC's structural changes was to move people out of poverty so that all children experience conditions that promote health, this policy agenda was difficult to achieve (Horsley & Ciske, 2005). PHSKC efforts target multiple SDOH intervention points, including economic opportunities, education, and childhood development.

The **Dudley Street Neighborhood Initiative (DSNI)** was created in 1984 out of residents' concerns about their community environment, from arson fires and illegal dumping (www.dsni.org/sustainable-economic-development). With support from the Mabel Louise Riley Foundation, an advisory group was created, and neighborhood revitalization plans were drawn up. In 1986, DSNI launched its first media campaign, "Don't Dump on Us," and from this DSNI cleaned vacant lots, eliminated illegal trash transfer stations, and created a land trust model. DSNI efforts addressed multiple SDOH, including housing, education, employment, physical environment, public safety, and the social environment. One of the main goals of DSNI was to empower residents of the community to change the conditions that they live in. Outcomes stemming from DSNI's efforts include increases in financial literacy, increased access to health care services, and improved education, exercise, and nutrition. DSNI targets education, housing, and the built environment as SDOH intervention points.

A leading health indicator in the US is educational achievement in adolescents. **Linked Learning** is a proven, systemic approach to education that helps students prepare for college and career, grow through real work experiences, and prepare to participate in civic life (www.linkedlearning.org/about/linked-learning-approach). Using rigorous academics, career technical education, work-based learning, and comprehensive support services, students succeed. Students in nine school districts that utilized Linked Learning over multiple years show that students are less likely to drop out, more likely to graduate, earn more credits by the end of high school, and build mindsets that help them thrive. Linked Learning targets SDOH intervention points of education and community cohesion.

Community gardens are one way to increase food access. Community gardens are pieces of land that are gardened and kept by groups of people, normally for home consumption rather than selling. Community gardens increase access to fruits and vegetables, increase fruit and vegetable consumption, and increase physical activity. One example of a community garden to promote health is the Yéego Gardening! intervention, designed to increase gardening behaviors, access low cost fruits and vegetables, and increase health food consumption in Navajo communities (Ornelas, Deschenie, Jim, et al., 2019). Gardens were created and maintained in partnership with community-based organizations in two communities. Monthly workshops during the growing season increased confidence and skills about gardening and healthy eating while teaching attendees about the Navajo culture. Results from the intervention demonstrate the importance of educational components and hands-on activities to impact social norms and healthy eating. Yéego Gardening! targets food access, nutrition, and community cohesion as SDOH intervention points.

Racism refers to organized systems within societies that cause avoidable and unfair inequalities in power, resources, capacities and opportunities across racial or ethnic groups (Paradies, Ben, Denson, et al., 2015). Racism may occur through beliefs, stereotypes, prejudices or discrimination. **Discrimination** refers to socially structured action that is unfair or unjustified and harms individuals and groups (Abramson, Hashemi, & Sánchez-Jankowski, 2015). We know that discrimination, unfair treatment, stigma, and racism occur at the individual and structural level. In Chapter 2 we reviewed unique populations that experience discrimination based on their race, ethnicity, gender, sexual orientation, and disability status. Discrimination can lead to long-term negative health outcomes. Globally, racism and discrimination are being viewed as targets for SDOH programming. The **ERASE Racism** organization leads public policy advocacy campaigns and related initiatives to promote racial equity in areas such as housing, public-school education, and community development in Long Island New York, and in regional, national partnerships. Their mission is to expose forms of racial discrimination, advocate for laws and policies that eliminate racial disparities, and increase understanding of how structural racism and segregation impact communities. Examples of their work cover inclusive housing, education equity, partnerships for racial equity, and civil rights monitoring (www.eraseracismny.org/about-us). ERASE Racism targets structural and systems bias as SDOH intervention points.

The **Greensboro Health Disparities Collaborative** was formed in 2003 when 25 community members, leaders, advocates, researchers, faculty, and health care professionals came together to understand and reduce racial and ethnic disparities. The Collaborative partnered with the People's Institute for Survival and Beyond to conduct an Undoing Racism workshop in the community. Later that year, members of the Collaborative signed a contract acknowledging the value of all people involved in the research process. In 2006, the Collaborative received a grant from the NIH for Cancer Care and Racial Equity Study (CCARES). This study sought to understand reasons for disparities between African American and White breast cancer patients (http://greensborohealth.org/index.html). Nettie Coad was a founding member of the Collaborative and, although she passed away in 2012, her vision for the Collaborative continues to build, drawing people and organizations together who have a common vision to improve health outcomes for everyone. The Collaborative targets structural and systems bias as SDOH intervention points.

Project Implicit, founded in 1998 by three scientists, is a non-profit organization and international collaboration between researchers who are interested in implicit social cognition—thoughts and feelings outside of conscious awareness and control (www.projectimplicit.net/). Implicit bias is unseen, unintentional, and unconscious. For example, implicit bias may occur due to a person's skin color or their accent. This type of bias influences how people are treated in health care, criminal justice settings, schools, and social service organizations (and more) (Blair, Steiner, & Havranek, 2011). Project Implicit's goal is to educate the public about hidden biases and to provide a "virtual laboratory" for collecting data on the Internet. Project Implicit Mental Health started in 2011 and provides diversity and inclusion training, leadership training, and consulting on how to apply the science of implicit bias and research findings into practice. Project Implicit targets structural and systems bias as intervention points.

Tebb and colleagues explored adolescent and young adult programs in a qualitative study with eight SDOH programs throughout the United States (Tebb, Pica, Twietmeyer, et al., 2018; and see Table 5.2).

Table 5.2 Examples of programs that address adolescent SDOH in the United States

Program	Description
The Los Angeles Trust for Children's Health, Los Angeles, CA	Student achievement by increasing access to integrated health care
One Degree, San Francisco, CA	Technology-driven organization linking low-income people with community resources
SHCIP, New Mexico and Colorado	Effective replicable strategies for enhancing health care quality
The Door, New York, NY	Comprehensive health and development services including reproductive health, mental health, legal assistance, educational support, college preparation, and English tutoring
Housing Rx, Boston, MA	Reduction of housing instability among low-income families with young children
Progreso Latino, Rhode Island	Latinos' and immigrants' access to free health care, dual-language adult education, and free/low-cost immigration legal services
Mount Sinai Adolescent Health Center, New York, NY	High-quality, comprehensive, confidential, and free health care to 24 middle- and high-school school-based health centers
Spartanburg County Community Indicators Project South Carolina, Spartanburg, SC	Health indicators, setting of improvement goals, and work with communities to coordinate improvements

Source: Tebb, Pica, Twietmeyer, et al. (2018).

Tebb and colleagues developed recommendations based on their review that may be useful as you develop, plan, implement, and evaluate programs using a SDOH lens. First, collaborate with multiple sectors of the community. Second, address the root causes of poverty through education, job training, and career pathways. Utilize a poverty focus with housing prescriptions and teen pregnancy prevention. Third, leverage technology in health to link care and community supports, and give access to a holistic system of care, informed by data-driven approaches. Fourth, address special populations, in this case adolescents and young adults, to address historical injustices through staffing and safe inclusive environments, and engage them in program activities. Fifth, advocate for public policies that address SDOH and seek flexible and diverse funding sources (Tebb et al., 2018).

Up until now we have reviewed program examples that have addressed SDOH and structural inequalities. Some are informed by evidence while other examples are building an evidence base through community best practices and programming. What might surprise you is that some policies and practices continue despite an evidence base that they do not work. One example is the Sex Offender Registration and Notification Act (SORNA), also known as the **Adam Walsh Child Protection and Safety Act of 2006** (see www.justice.gov/archive/olp/pdf/adam_walsh_act.pdf). SORNA requires that states maintain a registry of people convicted of sex offenses, expands the type of offenses for which a person must register, and applies to both adults and children (Justice Policy Institute, 2008). For example, Title 1 of the Adam Walsh Act includes the policy for juvenile sex offender registration and notification (JSORN). The implementation of JSORN is different in each state and has resulted in children as young as 9 years old being placed on a sex offender registry for decades to life (Pittman & Nguyen, 2011). What is most troubling about SORNA and JSORN is that guidelines have not changed despite repeated studies that show that registration and notification policies have no influence on sex crime rates (Levenson, Brannon, Fortney, et al., 2007). Further, placing children on sex offender registries has long-term and devastating impacts to the child, victim, family, and society at large. Although SORNA was designed to promote safety and reduce potential for abuse and harm, it has not achieved this.

The **Drug Abuse Resistance Education (DARE)** program is one of the most widely used programs in schools throughout the US. DARE was developed in 1983 by the Los Angeles Police Department and the Los Angeles School District. In 2001, DARE was offered in 80% of school districts throughout the US. Although there is significant evaluation evidence that DARE does not work, school districts and states continue to use it as their primary drug abuse prevention program. Evaluations consistently report positive effects immediately following participation in a program, but these impacts do not last as students become older (Birkeland, Murphy-Graham, & Weiss, 2005). In fact, evaluations indicate that there is no difference between students who participated in DARE and those who did not in later adolescence. Authors report that one of primary reasons that DARE continues in schools, despite the lack of evidence, is the relationship building that occurs between students and law enforcement. But federal legislation requires that school-based drug prevention programs are based on scientific evidence. Without scientific evidence, DARE will be hard pressed to continue. This is an example of a program that was designed with one goal, to prevent substance abuse. An evaluation that focuses on relationships, connections, and feelings of safety that come from the law enforcement–child interactions that occur through the DARE program could open the door for prevention programs that are backed by evidence.

With these SDOH program examples in mind, let's review examples of federal and private-sector SDOH programs and funding.

Federal programs and funding for SDOH

AmeriCorps **VISTA** is a program of the Corporation for National and Community Service (CNCS) that provides resources and staffing for organizations and agencies working to alleviate poverty and address poverty-related problems in local communities. AmeriCorps VISTA members are placed at sponsoring organizations and serve approximately 40 hours per week addressing issues which have been locally identified as community priorities. The project goals and activities are designed to build the sponsor's capacity to serve low-income communities (https://nationalservice.gov/documents/2019/fy20-annual-program-guidance-americorps-vista).

Administration for Children and Families (ACF) funds multiple programs serving families, children, individuals, and communities (www.acf.hhs.gov/grants). ACF grants are designed to support the economic and social well-being of families, children, individuals, and communities. Examples of ACF funding that aligns with a SDOH focus include head start programs, childcare, child support enforcement, community services, and refugee resettlement.

Centers for Disease Control and Prevention (CDC) drives population health efforts, and one example of a SDOH focused program it supports is the Achieving SDOH Population Improvement in Rural Environments (ASPIRE) award program. ASPIRE provides monetary awards for local health departments, recognizing excellence in rural communities that are committed to addressing the SDOH (www.naccho.org/programs/public-health-infrastructure/performance-improvement/community-health-assessment/hp2020-and-sdoh/social-determinants-of-health).

The **Environmental Protection Agency (EPA)** supports a variety of health research grant programs that include children's environmental health and disease prevention, healthy schools, and tribal health research agendas (www.epa.gov/research-grants/health-research-grants).

One example of a SDOH focused grant program is the **Housing and Urban Development (HUD)** Capacity Building (Section 4) Grants. The HUD Capacity Building for Community Development and Affordable Housing Program, commonly referred to as Section 4 supports SDOH programming efforts. Since Congressional authorization in 1993, the program has helped low-income families and neighborhoods in more than 2,000 urban and rural communities in all 50 states and the District of Columbia. HUD funds are used to build capacity and implement HUD programs, design, finance, and execute community development and affordable housing projects, coordinate on cross-programmatic, place-based approaches, and facilitate knowledge sharing (www.enterprisecommunity.org/financing-and-development/grants#section4).

The **National Cancer Institute (NCI) (NIH, US Department of Health and Human Services)** is improving the reach and quality of cancer care through several SDOH funding opportunities. One example is the Improving the Reach and Quality of Cancer Care in Rural Populations (https://grants.nih.gov/grants/guide/rfa-files/RFA-CA-19-064.html).

Examples of private-sector programming and funding

Most of the programs and examples in this text come from public and government funded initiatives to improve health. But private-sector funding for SDOH is beginning to take hold. Examples of private-sector SDOH programs that invest in population health come from corporate philanthropy, social/health entrepreneurship, and pay for success contracting (National Academies Press, 2016). Pay for success contracting focuses on upstream investments (prevention, programs, policy) that will reduce downstream costs to health and society.

The mission of the **Bill and Melinda Gates Foundation** in developing countries is to focus on improving people's health and well-being, helping individuals lift themselves out of hunger and extreme poverty. In the United States, the foundation works to ensure that all people—especially those with the fewest resources—can access the opportunities they need to succeed in school and life (Gates Foundation, 2019). Their mission in education, via the **High School Grants Initiative**, is to significantly increase the number of Black, Latino, and low-income students who earn a diploma, enroll in a postsecondary institution, and are on track in their first year to obtain a credential with labor-market value. The Gates Foundation's focus includes networks for school improvement, educator preparation, high quality charter schools, aligned instructional materials, social emotional learning, stronger pathways, and big bets in innovation (Gates Foundation, 2019).

> America's high schools are obsolete. By obsolete, I don't just mean that our high schools are broken, flawed, and under-funded—though a case could be made for every one of those points. By obsolete, I mean that our high schools—even when they're working exactly as designed—cannot teach our kids what they need to know today.... Today, only one-third of our students graduate from high school ready for college, work, and citizenship. The other two thirds, most of them low-income and minority students, are tracked into courses that won't ever get them ready for college or prepare them for a family-wage job—no matter how well the students learn, or the teachers teach. This isn't an accident or a flaw in the system; it is the system.
>
> (Bill & Melinda Gates Foundation, 2005)

Oprah Winfrey's leadership academy for girls was set up after she promised Nelson Mandela, the first president of post-apartheid South Africa, that she would build a boarding school for disadvantaged girls. These girls would become the next generation of leaders in South Africa. The $40 million dollar boarding school for girls in grades 7–12 sent out 5,500 application packs to girls from rural areas of South Africa. Of these 3,500 were returned with essays in which girls wrote about their dreams for the future. From these applications, 484 were selected for interviews and 152 were selected. Winfrey was criticized for money spent on the school facility and the limited reach that it would have into the needs of South Africa. Other critics felt her approach lacked a community basis, and that taking children away from their homes and communities was unethical. There will always be critics, but one topic that remains critical to the discussion is to explore the appropriate role of private philanthropy like Winfrey's, in relation to what is best for students, schools, and countries—and according to whom. When considering SDOH efforts, it is important to think about private resource allocation in a poor country, what kind of school is in the best interest of the students, and what kind of school is in the best interests of the country (Duke Sanford Center for Strategic Philanthropy and Civil Society, 2010).

Heifer International works in 21 countries around the world alongside local farmers and business owners (www.heifer.org/our-work/flagship-projects/east-africa-dairy-development-project.html). It supports farmers and communities as they mobilize and envision their futures, provides training so they can improve the quantity and quality of the goods they produce, and provides connections to market to increase sales and incomes. East Africa Dairy development is one Heifer project that is addressing limited food access through sustainable dairy markets. Heifer supported 230,000 dairy farmers to implement a sustainable system that would improve the quality and quantity of milk production, which would, in turn, allow farmers to borrow money against milk that had already been delivered, rather than waiting up to 90 days for payment. This 10-year project ended in 2018 and the impact is clear, African dairy farmers have increased incomes, higher yields on their farms, and long-term support to continue providing milk to families and countries throughout Africa. Heifer International targets food access, economic opportunities, and the built environment as SDOH intervention points.

The **Pew Research Center** is a non-profit, tax-exempt 501(c)3 organization and a subsidiary of The Pew Charitable Trusts, the primary funder of the Pew Research Center. The Center's empirically driven research on a wide range of topics helps key stakeholders in society—policymakers, media, and the public at large—understand and solve the world's most challenging problems. As a neutral source of data and analysis, Pew Research Center does not take policy positions. (www.pewtrusts.org/en/search?q=funding&sortBy=relevance&sortOrder=asc&page=1). It funds a variety of community, conservation, finance, governance, health, and related projects throughout the world. Its research and funding portfolio focuses on SDOH efforts and addressing health equity.

The **WK Kellogg Foundation** seeks to promote the health, happiness, and well-being of children. Kellogg funding supports thriving children, working families, and equitable communities. Kellogg builds health equity through connections with schools, childcare settings, professional environments, and communities (www.wkkf.org/grants). A review of its grant portfolio shows that since 2008 it has funded 20,763 grants to communities throughout the US. Priority locations include Michigan, Mississippi, New Mexico, New Orleans, Chiapas, and the Yucatan Peninsula in Mexico, and Central and South Haiti. One example of a Kellogg program that is addressing SDOH is the Family Engagement Cohort (2014–2017). Kellogg used a transformative family engagement framework to support cohort projects that would build institutional and system capacity and develop family leadership. Building institutional and system capacity involved addressing innate power dynamics, valuing parents as experts when it came to their children, integrating family, community, and culture into learning, and examining school communication to make it more effective. Developing family leadership efforts focused on building strong networks among families and communities, mobilizing skills to increase knowledge and control over resources, and helping families develop and assert leadership (Kellogg Foundation, 2019).

The **Robert Wood Johnson Foundation (RWJF)** is leading the way in SDOH program funding, evaluation, and dissemination efforts that build health equity for future generations. Its work focuses on healthy communities, healthy children, healthy weights, health leadership, and health systems. Within the healthy communities' focus, SDOH is a primary focus area. A brief review of the SDOH portfolio shows that RWJF has funded 7,312 projects totaling $3,316,665,775 across the globe (RWJF, 2019a). One of its funded grants addresses social isolation. Social networks can be protective against bullying, suicide, depression, and substance abuse among young people. RWJF funded several SDOH initiatives to address social isolation through ChangeX in Dublin, Ireland. ChangeX aims to empower communities to build a culture of health through innovative strategies. Other projects include:

- Building opportunities for physical activity in public places in 880 cities in the United States, Canada, and Nordic countries during the winter months
- Strengthening social networks in young people through organized sports, music, art, and dance, in the Matanuska Susitna Borough of Alaska
- Connecting families living in poverty to other social networks that build social inclusion while connecting them to food, job training, and housing assistance in Brazil
- Creating peer support networks for Latino Lesbian, Gay, Bisexual, Transgender, and Queer (LGBTQ) youth in Brazil, Peru, and a partnership with 4H clubs at Oregon State University
- Improving social connections for incarcerated citizen in the US so that they can form new relationships and maintain relationships with families, friends, and local community members in New Jersey, Connecticut, and Massachusetts

Summary

We began this chapter by exploring the cigarette epidemic and lung cancer. This narrative shows us the importance of understanding the role of people, policies, advertisements, and tobacco companies as contributors to the world's deadliest malignancy. Not just one person, place, policy, or thing created the lung cancer epidemic, and therefore not just one will solve the epidemic. We explored programs that address SDOH in a variety of settings, countries, and contexts. These programs represent different stream conditions, different needs, and different focus areas for SDOH efforts. RWJF is an excellent resource for evaluators and communities as they look toward action steps needed to improve health. Other resources with the CDC, and private, multisectoral collaborations will help with shifting public health programming toward a SDOH focus. What I find most inspiring about these programs is that they are effective, and because of multiple program efforts, stream conditions are changing, and health is improving at the population level.

Points to remember

1 Facts about SDOH have been established. Public health programs must address social determinants to improve population health.
2 There are 161 programs with scientific evidence that can be used to address upstream public health conditions. Many of these directly impact health disparities and health inequalities.
3 Other programs address SDOH but lack a scientific evidence base, though they may be just as effective as programs with an evidence base. Know the community, know the problem, and the desired outcomes.
4 Private-sector agents are funding SDOH efforts across the globe. Private-sector funders have more flexibility in how they address SDOH and often have more resources available.

Additional reading and resources

Centers for Disease Control and Prevention, Health in All Policies Guide for State and Local Governments
www.phi.org/uploads/application/files/udt4vq0y712qpb1o4p62dexjlgxlnogpq15gr8 pti3y7ckzysi.pdf

Racial Equity Resource Guide
www.racialequitytools.org/resourcefiles/Racial_Equity_Resource_Guide.pdf

Robert Wood Johnson Foundation's Take Action to Improve Health
www.countyhealthrankings.org/take-action-to-improve-health

United States Department of Agriculture Food Deserts
www.ers.usda.gov/data-products/food-access-research-atlas/documentation/

Chapter questions

1   Review Wilkinson and Marmot's 10 solid facts that we started this chapter with. These were published in 2003, so how have the field and SDOH facts evolved since that time?
2   What are the differences between racism and discrimination? How do these relate to individual and population health?
3   Describe food access, food utilization, and food availability as they relate to health. How does low-income status impact one's ability to access food?
4   Summarize how private organizations are leading SDOH programming efforts in the United States and World. What are some of the criticism of these approaches?
5   Discuss the importance of involving underserved and underrepresented populations in SDOH programming.

Activities on the web

1   Go to https://implicit.harvard.edu/implicit/ and complete their surveys on social attitudes, project implicit health, and project implicit featured task for random topics. What did you learn about yourself in this process? How do you think implicit bias relates to SDOH and PHE?
2   Visit the Robert Wood Johnson Foundation SDOH webpage. Review featured initiatives. Select one initiative and write about why and how this initiative addresses SDOH. Discuss any gaps in the initiative and add considerations for SDOH focused evaluation.

References

Abramson, C. M., Hashemi, M., & Sánchez-Jankowski, M. (2015). Perceived discrimination in US healthcare: Charting the effects of key social characteristics within and across racial groups. *Preventive Medicine Reports*, (2), 615–621. doi.org/10.1016/j.pmedr.2015.07.006.

American Academy of Family Physicians. (2018). *Health Care for All: A framework for moving to a primary care-based health care system in the United States*. Retrieved from: www.aafp.org/about/policies/all/health-care-for-all.html.

Bill & Melinda Gates Foundation. (2005). National Education Summit speech. Available from: www.gatesfoundation.org/media-center/speeches/2005/02/bill-gates-2005-national-education-summit.

Birkeland, S., Murphy-Graham, E., & Weiss, C. (2005). Good reasons for ignoring good evaluation: The case of the drug abuse resistance education (DARE) program. *Evaluation and Program Planning*, 28(3), 247–256.

Blair, I. V., Steiner, J. F., & Havranek, E. P. (2011). Unconscious (implicit) bias and health disparities: Where do we go from here? *The Permanente Journal*, 15(2), 71–78.

Centers for Disease Control and Prevention. (2019). *Health Impact in 5 Years Project*. Retrieved from: www.cdc.gov/policy/hst/hi5/index.html.

Chriqui, J. F., Taber, D. R., Slater, S. J., Turner, L., Lowrey, K. M., & Chaloupka, F. J. (2012). The impact of state safe routes to school-related laws on active travel to school policies and practices in US elementary schools. *Health & Place*, 18(1), 8–15.

Cowan, D., Hubsmith, D., & Ping, R. (2011). Safe routes to school local policy guide. Available from: www.saferoutespartnership.org/sites/default/files/pdf/Local_Policy_Guide_2011.pdf.

Duke Sanford Center for Strategic Philanthropy and Civil Society. (2010). An inspired model or a misguided one? Oprah Winfrey's dream school for impoverished South African girls. Retrieved from: https://cspcs.sanford.duke.edu/learning-resources/case-study-database/inspired-model-or-misguided-one-oprah-winfrey-s-dream-school.

Gates Foundation (2019). K-12 education strategy: Goals and area of focus. Retrieved from: www.gatesfoundation.org/What-We-Do/US-Program/K-12-Education.

Harris, A. D., McGregor, J. C., Perencevich, E. N., Furuno, J. P., Zhu, J., Peterson, D. E., & Finkelstein, J. (2006). The use and interpretation of quasi-experimental studies in medical informatics. *Journal of the American Medical Informatics Association: JAMIA, 13*(1), 16–23. doi:10.1197/jamia.M1749.

Horsley, K., & Ciske, S. J. (2005). From neurons to King County neighbourhoods: Partnering to promote policies based on the science of early childhood development. *American Journal of Public Health, 95*(4), 562–567.

Institute of Medicine (2014). Population health implications of the Affordable Care Act: Workshop summary. Retrieved from https://ebookcentral.proquest.com.

Institute of Medicine and National Research Council. (2000). *From neurons to neighbourhoods: The science of early childhood development.* Washington, DC: The National Academies Press. doi:10.17226/9824.

Justice Policy Institute. (2008). *Registering harm: How sex offense registries fail youth communities.* Available from: www.justicepolicy.org/research/1939.

Kelley, A. (2018). *Evaluation in rural communities.* London: Routledge. doi:10.4324/9780429458224.

Kellogg Foundation (2019). *Cultivating a community of champions for children through transformative family engagement.* Retrieved from: www.wkkf.org/resource-directory.

Levenson, J. S., Brannon, Y. N., Fortney, T., & Baker, J. (2007). Public perceptions about sex offenders and community protection policies. *Analyses of Social Issues and Public Policy, 7*(1), 137–161.

Melkas, T. (2013). Health in all policies as a priority in Finnish health policy: A case study on national health policy development. *Scandinavian Journal of Public Health, 41*(11, Suppl.), 3–28. doi:10.1177/1403494812472296.

National Academies Press (2016). Applying a health lens to business practices, policies, and investments: Workshop summary. Washington, DC: National Academies Press. Retrieved from: www.nap.edu/read/21842/chapter/1.

Ornelas, I. J., Deschenie, D., Jim, J., Bishop, S., Lombard, K., & Beresford, S. A. (2017). Yéego Gardening! A community garden intervention to promote health on the Navajo Nation. *Progress in Community Health Partnerships: Research, Education, and Action, 11*(4), 417–425. doi:10.1353/cpr.2017.0049.

Paradies, Y., Ben, J., Denson, N., Elias, A., Priest, N., Pieterse, A., ... & Gee, G. (2015). Racism as a determinant of health: A systematic review and meta-analysis. *PLoS ONE, 10*(9), e0138511. doi:10.1371/journal.pone.0138511.

Pittman, N., & Nguyen, Q. (2011). *A snapshot of juvenile sex offender registration and notification laws: A survey of the United States.* Philadelphia, PA: Defender Association of Philadelphia. Retrieved from www.njjn.org/uploads/digital-library/SNAPSHOT_web10-28.pdf.

Plucinski, M. (2016). Health in all policies: Sacred traditional tobacco for healthy Native communities. American Indian Cancer Foundation. Retrieved from: www.preventcancer.org/wp-content/uploads/2016/04/Melanie-Plucinski-Dialogue-2016-2.pdf.

Proctor, R. (2012). The history of the discovery of the cigarette–lung cancer link: Evidentiary traditions, corporate denial, global toll. *Tobacco Control*, *21*(2), 87–91.

Puska, P. (2006). Health in all policies. *The European Journal of Public Health*, *17*(4), 328.

Rice, W. R. (1989). Analyzing tables of statistical tests. *Evolution*, *43*(1), 223–225.

Robert Wood Johnson Foundation (2019a). Grants explorer, Healthy Communities, social determinants of health. Retrieved from: www.rwjf.org/en/how-we-work/grants-explorer. html#t=1930.

Robert Wood Johnson Foundation (2019b). Policies and programs that improve health. Scientifically supported. Retrieved from: www.countyhealthrankings.org/take-action-to-improve-health/what-works-for-health/policies?f%5B0%5D=field_program_evidence_rating%3A1.

Tebb, K. P., Pica, G., Twietmeyer, L., Diaz, A., & Brindis, C. D. (2018). Innovative approaches to address social determinants of health among adolescents and young adults. *Health Equity*, *2*(1), 321–328. doi:10.1089/heq.2018.0011.

Wilkinson, R. G., & Marmot, M. (Eds.). (2003). Social determinants of health: The solid facts. World Health Organization. Retrieved from: https://books.google.com/books?hl=en&lr=&id=QDFzqNZZHLMC&oi=fnd&pg=PA5&dq=marmot+and+wilkinson+2003&ots=xVuJfBURju&sig=vgWIEX1gQapfhyZaHYcydGGFkCM#v=onepage&q=marmot%20and%20wilkinson%202003&f=false.

6   SDOH evaluation examples

Learning objectives

After reading this chapter, you should be able to:

- List examples of upstream, midstream, and downstream evaluations
- Describe evaluation targets for each of the SDOH targets
- Explain why some SDOH evaluations document impact while others do not
- Discuss policy change as an upstream evaluation target and provide examples of how policy change impacts health equity and empowerment

One of the defining characteristics of a SDOH evaluation is the focus on health equity—meaning that everyone has fair, equal, and just opportunities to be as healthy as they possibly can. As you might recall from previous chapters, evaluation is the examination of the worth, merit, or significance of an object. Objects may be programs, with specific goals and objectives, interventions, research initiatives, advocacy and campaign efforts, or training programs (CDC, 2012). As we review examples of SDOH evaluations from the literature, let's consider the stream locations, SDOH pathways, and potential indicators shown in Table 6.1.

In the next sections we will explore SDOH program examples. You will observe that many of these program evaluations did not include SDOH terms, but their focus on health equity and structural determinants indicates a SDOH focused evaluation is appropriate. Table 6.2 summarizes SDOH program examples, structural determinants, SDOH pathways, and potential indicators.

> *I have a home after 39 years of living on the streets … it takes me a long time to get here, to the shelter for food. They check on you … make sure that you aren't drinking or doing drugs. I have to keep clean you know. I feel different living there. I don't know if it is just the walls or if it is just me.*

This is the story from a 75-year-old Vietnam veteran. How did having a place to live, a permanent house, improve his quality of life? His health and longevity? His sense of community? His sobriety? His access to equal, just, and fair health? As evaluators of SDOH programs we must consider the lives

Table 6.1 Stream locations, SDOH pathways, and indicators

Stream Location & Desired Conditions	SDOH Pathway	Indicators
Upstream—All people and all communities live in communities that support fair, equal, and just opportunities for health	Structural Inequities	Change in: socioeconomic context and position, differential exposure, differential vulnerability, differential health care, and differential consequences
	Institutional Power	Change in: corporations, businesses, government, schools, laws and regulations, policies
Midstream—Move people to conditions that support health and well-being	Living Conditions Community Conditions	Improvements in: good paying jobs, quality education, access to health care, access to transportation, access to physical activity
Downstream—Change behaviors or conditions that cause poor health	Risk Behaviors Risk Conditions	Reduced: smoking, poor nutrition, limited physical activity, obesity, homelessness, low birth weight, untreated mental illness, violence, alcohol and other drugs, sexual behaviors, poor health status
	Disease and Injury	Reduced: communicable disease, chronic disease, injuries

Considerations of Policy, Community Capacity, and Civic Engagement also need to be included in a SDOH.

Table 6.2 Chapter examples, SDOH pathways, and indicators/results

Chapter 6 Program Example	SDOH Pathway	Indicators
Human Impact Youth Diversion Program (Human Impact Partners, 2019)	Structural inequalities	Racial equity, % of youth stops by race and ethnicity, comparison of youth racial identity in the population, review stops, disproportionate contacts in specific neighborhoods.
Mass Incarceration Policy Change (Acker, Braveman, Arkin, et al., 2019).	Structural inequalities	Incarceration and crime rates, sentencing length, policy change, power sharing
Well London Study (Wall, Hayes, Moore, et al., 2009)	Structural inequalities, living conditions, community conditions, risk behaviors and conditions	Participation of vulnerable populations, healthy eating, physical activity, general health, and mental well-being
TransForm Baltimore (Thornton Greiner, Fichtenberg, et al., 2013)	Structural inequalities, living conditions, community conditions	Revised zoning rules, improved living conditions, reductions in crime, improved physical health
Medicaid 1115 Waiver (North Carolina Department of Health and Human Services, 2018)	Structural inequalities, institutional power, disease and injury	Participation of vulnerable populations, change in policies and power, quality education, health care access, transport, physical activity
Maternal Infant and Early Childhood Home Visiting Program (HRSA, 2019)	Structural inequalities, living conditions, risk behaviors, risk conditions	Participation of vulnerable populations, early screening and referral for physical, behavioral, or mental health needs, increases school readiness, reduce intimate partner violence, and increase parent-child attachment
Drug Treatment Courts (Rezansoff, Moniruzzaman, Clark, et al., 2015)	Structural inequalities, living and community conditions	Participation of vulnerable populations, change in laws and policies, improvement to health and access services, reductions in risk behaviors, conditions, and disease/injury

continued

Table 6.2 continued

Chapter 6 Program Example	SDOH Pathway	Indicators
Healthy Cities Movement (Norris & Pittman, 2000)	Structural inequalities – living and community conditions, risk behaviors	Participation of vulnerable populations, community involvement, improve living and community conditions, reductions in risk and behavior conditions
Tribal Prevention Initiative (Kelley, Witzel, & Fatupaito, 2019).	Structural inequalities	Participation of vulnerable populations, improved community conditions, reduced risk behaviors
Intergenerational Connections Project (Kelley, Small, Small, et al., 2018)	Structural inequalities, community conditions	Change in community conditions that support cultural resilience, reduced risk behaviors and conditions
Transitional Recovery and Culture Project (Kelley, Bingham, Brown, et al., 2017).	Structural inequalities, community conditions, risk behaviors	Participation of vulnerable populations, increased access to health care and treatment, change in norms/stigma around addiction, reduced risk behaviors and reduced disease and injury
Healthy Kids, Healthy Communities (RWJF, 2014)	Institutional power, living and community conditions	Changes in policy system to improve healthy eating and active living, reduced risk behaviors and conditions, reduced childhood obesity

of people. We cannot assume we know what is best or what will improve someone's health and quality of life. If we keep our eyes on empowerment as an end goal of SDOH programming, then we can see that there are many different ways that this occurs. Empowerment does not just happen through gaining material resources, but in access to power in relation to the world around us.

Upstream policy and special populations

Human Impact Youth Diversion Program (HIP). In 2017, Los Angeles County established an Office of Youth Diversion and Development to advance a collaboratively designed pre-booking diversion initiative that prevents youth from getting formally arrested. This also included youth who were referred to probation during encounters with law enforcement. Human Impact Partners and the Los Angeles (LA) County Office of Youth Diversion and Development (YDD) worked collaboratively to develop an evaluation framework that would assess and prevent racial inequities in this program (https://humanimpact.org/hipprojects/evaluateyouthdiversion/). We know from previous chapters that definitions are important, so let's review these now. **Diversion** is a promising practice for reducing youth involvement with the justice system. Unfortunately, research indicates that when programs fail to promote equity in how they are designed and implemented, they create more racial inequity (Human Impact Partners, 2019). There are multiple ways in which diversion can happen, but HIP focuses on community-based, pre-booking diversion for youth. HIP identified five main touch points in pre-booking diversions: getting stopped by a law enforcement official, getting referred by law enforcement to a diversion program, getting enrolled in a diversion program, participating and completing a program, and thriving in the program. **Racial equity** is both an outcome and a process. The Center for Social Inclusion defines it this way:

> Racial equity is about applying justice and a little bit of common sense to a system that's been out of balance. When a system is out of balance, people of color feel the impacts most acutely, but to be clear, an imbalanced system makes all of us pay.

> (Center for Social Inclusion, nd, p. 1)

This evaluation measured outcomes of Black and Brown youth at each of the five touch points listed previously and compared them with White youth. LA County and HIP developed promising practices to reduce racial inequities across all touch points, these including: creation of collaborative decision-making structures that focus on Black and Brown youth voices and that grow leadership skills, investment in sustainable resources, reduction of burdens on youth and caretakers, and tracking and ensuring protected access to data.

Another example from HIP is the **Stopwatch program**. This occurred in Boston from 2004–2006. Stopwatch provided training on trauma, youth development, implicit bias, and cultural humility for transportation authority police—youth arrests on the subway went from 680 in 2001 to 84 in 2009 (Rosenbaum & Lawrence, 2011).

Mass incarceration policy change. A major shift in mass incarceration practices is needed in the United States. It is as an issue of health equity, and therefore an appropriate SDOH focus for evaluation. With approximately 2.2 million US adults and youth behind bars, the United States incarcerates many more persons—both in absolute numbers and as a percentage of the population—than any other nation in the world (Acker, Braveman, Arkin, et al., 2019). Results from RWJF efforts show that mass incarceration negatively impacts everyone's health and well-being at the social, educational, economic, and emotional levels, with decreased life expectancy and greater prevalence of chronic health problems. Impacts extend to children of parents who are incarcerated, and to people of color, people with disabilities, and people with lower socioeconomic status. RWJF calls attention to inequitable policies and practices like mandatory minimal sentencing, three strikes provision, and high rates of incarceration among vulnerable communities and places. RWJF investigated states that have passed laws intended to reduce incarceration and crime rates simultaneously, such as reducing excessively long sentences—these states have reduced incarceration and crime. The First Step Act (see https://fas.org/sgp/crs/misc/R45558.pdf) was enacted December 21, 2018 and has the potential to reach 180,000 Americans in federal prisons. But a key issue is that this Act does not address the SDOH or the primary drivers of mass incarceration. This is an example of how an evaluation can explore existing laws and policies that impact health and build health equity upstream.

The **Well London Study** (Wall, Hayes, Moore, et al., 2009) was financed by the Big Lottery "Well-being" Fund and implemented by a consortium of London-based agencies led by the Greater London Authority and the London Health Commission. Well London implemented a set of complex interventions across 20 deprived areas of London that focused on healthy eating, healthy physical activity, and mental health and well-being. Interventions were designed and executed with community participation. Their approach included a randomized study design with an intervention and control group, designed to provide an overall assessment of the Well London objectives, and critical path analyses that could inform future replication in other communities. Results from the Well London evaluation show there was no evidence of impact on the primary outcomes of healthy eating, physical activity, general health, and mental well-being. Potential reasons for the lack of evidence may be related to low participation rates, changes in population, and sampling bias. Authors of this study call for improved methods that explore longitudinal pathways of health interventions and outcomes, along with theories of change that support pathways selected. Not all programs will result in a desired change in health outcome, but the Well London Study is an important step toward building health equity because of its focused interventions on 20 deprived areas across London. This is an example of an upstream SDOH evaluation that targeted class, race/ethnicity, and geographic location.

The goal of **Transform Baltimore** was to improve population health through changes to Baltimore's zoning code (Thornton, Greiner, Fichtenberg, et al., 2013). Team members used a health impact assessment (HIA) process to explore Baltimore's zoning code and revise it to impact health outcomes of physical activity, violent crime, and obesity. Using key informant interviews and existing literature as a guide, the authors estimated the potential impacts in high- and low-poverty neighborhoods for revisions in zoning. Results from this effort show the importance of upstream zoning and policy change to improve environmental conditions that impact health. The authors report that if zoning was revised, the percentage of people living in districts that allowed for mixed use and off-premise alcohol outlets would increase three-fold, less than 20% would live in districts that had new transit-oriented development zones, and all residents would live in places with lighting and landscaping guidelines (Thornton et al., 2013).

Medicaid programs serve more than 75 million Americans who experience low income. They are considered vulnerable populations whose health is often most negatively impacted by social determinants, such as lack of quality afford-able housing, food, and transportation. Medicaid Section 1115 demonstration waivers offer states freedom to try new approaches to administering Medicaid programs that depart from existing federal rules yet are consistent with the overall goals of the program. Evaluation of the impact of Medicaid 1115 waivers is under way (www.medicaid.gov/medicaid-chip-program-information/by-topics/waivers/1115/downloads/evaluation-design.pdf). States like North Carolina are receiving waivers and federal approval to implement the transition to Medicaid managed care and integrate physical health, behavioral health, and pharmacy benefits. Waivers allow for managed care plans and support the Healthy Opportunities pilot program designed to improve health and reduce health care costs (North Carolina Department of Health and Human Services, 2018). The Medicaid 1115 wavier is an example of policy and systems change to support health equity in populations throughout the United States. It is too soon to tell if these waivers and this new-found freedom have had a positive impact on health equity—continued evaluation of this and other upstream approaches are needed to improve health for all.

The **Maternal Infant and Early Childhood Home Visiting program (MIECHV)** is an evidence-based program that funds home visiting for at-risk preg-nant women and parents with children under the age of 5. The Health Services Administration (HRSA) and Administration for Children and Families fund MIECHV programs in states, tribal nations, and territories throughout the US. In 2018 alone they allocated $400 million over the year to support evidence-based home visiting models. Home visiting is an upstream approach that targets positive parenting skills, early learning and communication, information about health-related topics, screenings, and connecting families to additional services when needed (https://mchb.hrsa.gov/sites/default/files/mchb/MaternalChildHealthInitiatives/Home Visiting/pdf/programbrief.pdf). MIECHV efforts target families living below the federal poverty level, families with less than a high school education, and families that rely on Medicaid or the Child Health Insurance Program. Evaluation results show that MIECHV is effective in improving the well-being of parents and children throughout their lifespan:

- 70% of children enrolled in MIECHV report having family members that read to them, told them stories, or sang to them.
- 74% of children received timely screening for developmental delays.
- 92% of caregivers were asked if they had behavioral, developmental, or learning concerns.
- 82% of caregivers were screened for intimate partner violence.
- 78% of caregivers were screened for depression (HRSA, 2019).

MIECHV home visiting programs and evaluation efforts target multiple structural and SDOH pathways that improve health equity and health outcomes in vulnerable populations.

Midstream

Our physical environment, social environment, economic and work environment, and service environment shape health. Here are some examples of SDOH evaluations that address midstream determinants.

Drug Treatment Courts (DTCs) reduce the likelihood of substance-related criminal recidivism and are based on a coordinated response from judges, prosecutors and defense attorneys, probation authorities, and other stakeholders. A key feature of DTCs is that they adjudicate dockets of selected, non-violent substance-dependent offenders who have agreed to court-monitored substance use treatment rather than incarceration (Rezansoff, Moniruzzaman, Clark, et al., 2015). SDOH literature describes the relationship between criminal offending and social inequalities. Evaluation results from one DTC show that participants increased engagement with community-based health services and social services. Women with a mental disorder and concurrent disorders were more likely to use mental health and social services than men. The authors of this study call for evaluation of the SDOH in offender and rehabilitation crime reduction programs. SDOH focused evaluation targets include social support, social and occupational functioning, financial and child support, educational opportunities, and employment.

We can explore how drug court services could potentially address SDOH domains. Take a look at Table 6.3.

The **Healthy Cities Movement** was designed in the 1987 by WHO to improve the quality of life in 34 European cities. This movement was designed to change environments to support health and prevent disease through networks and organizations that build community (Wadell, 1995). The United States followed suit and began health community partnerships with health care organizations, public health organizations, cities, foundations, and civic organizations. In the United States, the Healthy Cities Movement aimed to engage diverse partners toward a shared vision that would result in multisectoral change.

Table 6.3 SDOH pathway, drug court services, and indicators example

SDOH Pathway	Drug Court Services	Indicators
Neighborhood living conditions	Residential treatment, drug free housing, housing vouchers	% of participants placed, number living in drug free housing, number and use of housing vouchers
Opportunities for learning and development	GED classes, completion, family skill building, supervised visitation with children	% of participants enrolled in GED classes, number completing family skill building, number of supervised visits
Community development and employment opportunities	Transitional employment and job training	% of participants in employment and job training, increases in community and employment opportunities
Social cohesion, civic engagement, and collective efficacy	Judge is a team leader, civil proceeding, review hearings, accountability and drug testing, community volunteer hours as a sanction, and fundraising marches	Justice, fairness, racial equity, number of hours worked in community, % of negative drug tests, funds raised, sustainability efforts visible

One example from the Healthy Cities Movement is the Bethel New Life partnership in Chicago, Illinois. This partnership, led by the Bethel New Life Baptist Church, has a vision to create a safe, affordable, and just community. Business leaders and communities of faith come together to address environmental issues, lack of jobs, and poor housing while promoting the overall well-being of African Americans living in low-income neighborhoods (Flower, 1996).

Evaluation results from the Healthy Cities Movement identified seven characteristics of a healthy community.

1 Practices ongoing dialogue among residents to build relationships and a shared vision of what the community is, what it should be, and how to get there
2 Generates leadership within the community, fosters a leadership style that emphasizes facilitation and collaboration, and encourages coalitions and partnerships
3 Shapes its future based on a shared vision of the community
4 Embraces the diversity of its residents
5 Gathers information about its assets and needs
6 Connects people to community resources
7 Creates a sense of responsibility and belonging among its residents (Norris & Pittman, 2000, p. 121)

The Healthy Cities Movement has reached more than 3,000 communities in more than 50 countries on every continent (Norris & Pittman, 2000). Evaluation of the Healthy Cities Movement shows that it is a challenge, as "after 20 years, many key dilemmas constantly reappear, people often looking for a kind of 'magic' list of universally applicable indicators to evaluate these initiatives" (O'Neill & Simard, 2006, p. 145). Leaders of the movement call for a change in how community members and practitioners address the symptoms of social problems and the underlying cultures that cause disease. The Healthy Cities Movement indirectly reaches all SDOH evaluation targets.

Mid and downstream social support and community cohesion

We know from early work on the SDOH that social exclusion, lack of social support, and limited community cohesion places people at risk for a variety of health problems (Wilkinson & Marmot, 2003). A multitude of programs throughout the world are building social support and community cohesion to address mid and downstream health inequalities, disparities, and inequities.

The **Tribal Prevention Initiative (TiPI)** addressed limited prosocial activities in communities through tribal best practices and documenting the relationship between social support, community connections, self-esteem, and culture on misuse in American Indian youth (Kelley, Witzel, & Fatupaito, 2019). TiPI was developed in response to tribal leaders voicing concerns about the lack of prevention activities available and the high prevalence of substance use among youth. Many youths did not have opportunities to learn about their culture, histories, and languages because of the disintegration of family units due to drugs, alcohol, and family member incarceration. Although the goal of the project was to reduce binge drinking in youth by 30% and increase community readiness by one overall point, the project did much more. It helped document the associations between participation in cultural activities, feelings of cultural and community connections, and decreased substance use. By providing opportunities for cultural involvement, youth protective factors increased, and risk factors associated with alcohol decreased (Kelley, Witzel, & Fatupaito, 2019). Evaluation results show that when youth were connected to their community, they were less likely to use marijuana. Similarly, when youth reported higher levels of social support, they were less likely to report drug and alcohol use. TiPI is an example of a midstream and downstream intervention that addresses multiple SDOH evaluation targets including midstream targets such as physical environment and social environment, and downstream targets like alcohol and drug use.

Cultural resilience and the Intergenerational Connections Project (ICP). Native American youth are placed at greater risk for suicide than any other age or ethnic population in the United States. Cultural resilience is a protective factor that has helped Native Americans overcome adversity. Intergenerational mentoring can moderate or reduce these risk factors. The ICP facilitated by Native PRIDE works with advisory councils in four Native communities in

Montana and South Dakota to build individual and community cultural resilience. Evaluation of ICP focuses on how communities define cultural resilience and how cultural resilience can be operationalized in a cultural context. ICP developed a cultural resilience scale that was administered at the beginning of the project and six months later, at the end of the project. Evaluation results show that cultural resilience increased significantly for all scale items. Community definitions include terms related to adversity and the transfer of cultural knowledge through sharing, participation, and involvement. Interviews with community members, elders, and youth underscore the importance of spirituality, language, values, and interactions between elders and youth. Evaluation results provide evidence that intergenerational mentoring opportunities can build community resilience, and help communities address high rates of suicide in Native communities (Kelley, Small, Small, et al., 2018). ICP addressed SDOH evaluation targets of, midstream, social and cultural environment, and, downstream, risk behaviors.

The **Transitional Recovery and Culture Project** (TRAC) was a six-year project that provided peer recovery support services (PRS) for individuals in recovery from substance use disorders. TRAC's SDOH focus addressed the lack of recovery supports in communities and issues of discrimination and racism within health care and treatment facilities, housing providers, and other social services institutions. PRS is based on the lived experience of recovery and provides a non-clinical recovery support environment for individuals to recover and heal. By providing opportunities for peers to meet with other peers with the lived experiences of recovery, this decreased substance use, and increased well-being, quality of life, and satisfaction with relationships among family and friends (Kelley, Bingham, Brown, et al., 2017). Evaluation results from the TRAC project show that PRS decreased substance use, increased help-seeking behaviors, and improved relationships between family and friends. TRAC efforts increased community awareness about addiction as a disease and decreased stigma associated with seeking help and treatment within the community and among providers. TRAC addressed several SDOH evaluation targets including social environment, physical environment, and downstream risk behaviors of alcohol and other drug use.

Healthy Kids, Healthy Communities is a national program funded by RWJF. The goal of this program was to prevent childhood obesity in 49 community partnerships across the United States. Key findings from this evaluation show that community partnerships generated more than $137,390,495 in matching funds. A total of 616 assessments were conducted in all program sites, with half exploring active living and the other half exploring healthy eating. Evaluation methods were designed to assess policy, system, and environmental changes as a result of the community partnerships' efforts to increase healthy eating and active living to reduce childhood obesity. Priority evaluation strategies were at the community and childcare/after-school level. Other strategies of interest include joint use, safe routes to school, zoning, comprehensive learning, grocery stories, nutrition assistance, and gardens and green houses. The most common changes identified in the evaluation were policy, practice, and environmental changes that were nutrition related. The second most common change was physical activity in childcare settings (RWJF, 2014). Healthy Kids, Healthy Communities addressed SDOH evaluation targets of physical environment, social environment, and downstream risk behaviors of poor nutrition and limited physical activity.

Summary

In this chapter we have explored SDOH evaluation program examples that address the SDOH at the upstream, midstream, and downstream locations. We explored structural inequalities and the SDOH pathway that creates conditions for poor health. Evaluation of programs follows a natural progression of exploring the impact of SDOH interventions on intended outcomes, vulnerable populations, and building health equity. We began this chapter exploring stream locations, SDOH domains, and program indicators. Then we reviewed the powerful work at the Human Impact Project to build racial equity for youth. Next, we explored midstream program evaluations from DTCs to efforts that build social support and community cohesion. We finished this chapter with a look at mid- and downstream evaluations and the Healthy Kids, Healthy Communities program. From this and other evaluations we can see there are challenges and strengths in each SDOH evaluation selected. What is important is that we learn from these examples and get a better idea about what SDOH evaluations look like and the kinds of data, metrics, and results we can expect.

Points to remember

1   There are multiple examples of programs focusing on evidence-based determinants of health. Some are more effective than others.
2   Knowing the stream location is important for program evaluation. Evaluation targets depend on them—consider social inequities, institutional power, living conditions, and risk behaviors as a start.
3   Evaluation of SDOH programs may not result in desired outcomes. Remember the Well London study? Even though this is the case, it does not mean that we should abandon efforts to evaluate them.
4   We can learn a lot about SDOH programs through evaluation. Consider multiple levels of evaluation, different metrics, and equity in the planning and implementation process.
5   Finally, programs may be political in nature, drawing criticism from both sides about the ethical dilemmas associated with working in developing countries, rich vs. poor, and more.

Additional reading and resources

Human Impact Partners
https://humanimpact.org/

Medicaid Innovation and SDOH
www.medicaidinnovation.org/_images/content/2019-IMI-Social_Determinants_
of_Health_in_Medicaid-Report.pdf

Chapter questions

1   Describe the stream locations, SDOH domains, and program evaluation targets presented in Table 6.1.
2   Summarize one program evaluation example from each of the streams, upstream, midstream, and downstream.
3   What are seven characteristics of a healthy community as defined by the Healthy Cities Movement? How do these relate to SDOH?
4   List three examples of upstream program evaluation approaches that resulted in health equity.
5   How do program examples in this chapter empower people and communities? Are there aspects of programs that may be disempowering? Discuss this and approaches to promote equitable distribution of power in health programs and policy making.

Activities on the web

1   Search the web for evaluation of SDOH programs. Identify three program evaluations that included SDOH from each of the stream locations (upstream, midstream, and downstream).
2   Review the Human Impact Project evaluation design (https://humanimpact. org/hipprojects/evaluateyouthdiversion/). List the metrics they used to document racial equity. What are the five touch points and what metrics did they use to document impact? List additional metrics that might be used.
3   Search the web for policies that were developed based on a SDOH evaluation and evidence base. Select one and provide an overview of the policy, location, target population, and impact on health equity.

References

Acker, J., Braveman, P., Arkin, E., Leviton, L., Parsons, J., & Hobor, G. (2018). *Mass incarceration threatens health equity in America*. Robert Wood Johnson Foundation. Retrieved from: www.rwjf.org/en/library/research/2019/01/mass-incarceration-threatens-health-equity-in-america.html.
Center for Social Inclusion. (nd). What is racial equity? Glenn Harris, President CSI. Retrieved from: www.centerforsocialinclusion.org/our-work/what-is-racial-equity/.
Centers for Disease Control and Prevention. (2012). Evaluation guide resources index. Retrieved from: www.cdc.gov/eval/guide/resources/index.htm.
Flower, J. (1996). *Bethel New Life, Chicago: A case study of community transformation*. The Healthcare Forum, Leadership Strategies for Health Care. Available from: https:// people.well.com/user/bbear/bethel.html.

Health Resources Services Administration. (2019). Maternal Child Health Initiatives Home Visiting Program brief. Retrieved from: https://mchb.hrsa.gov/sites/default/files/mchb/MaternalChildHealthInitiatives/HomeVisiting/pdf/programbrief.pdf.

Human Impact Partners. (2019). *Advancing racial Equity in youth diversion: An evaluation framework informed by Los Angeles county*. Available from: https://humanimpact.org/hipprojects/evaluateyouthdiversion/.

Kelley, A., Bingham, D., Brown, E., & Pepion, L. (2017). Assessing the impact of American Indian peer recovery support on substance use and health. *Journal of Groups in Addiction & Recovery, 12*(4), 296–308.

Kelley, A., Small, C., Small, M. C., Montileaux, H., & White, S. (2018). Defining cultural resilience to strengthen Native youth: A brief report from the Intergenerational Connection Project. *Practicing Anthropology, 40*(4), 5–9. doi:10.17730/0888-4552.40.4.5.

Kelley, A., Witzel, M., & Fatupaito, B. (2019). Preventing substance use in American Indian youth: The case for social support and community connections. *Substance Use & Misuse, 54*(5), 787–795. doi:10.1080/10826084.2018.1536724.

North Carolina Department of Health and Human Services. (2018). North Carolina receives 1115 Waiver approval, a major milestone for Medicaid and NC health care system. Retrieved from: www.ncdhhs.gov/news/press-releases/north-carolina-receives-1115-waiver-approval-major-milestone-medicaid-and-nc.

Norris, T., & Pittman, M. (2000). The healthy communities movement and the coalition for healthier cities and communities. *Public Health Reports, 115*(2–3), 118.

O'Neill, M., & Simard, P. (2006). Choosing indicators to evaluate Healthy Cities projects: A political task? *Health Promotion International, 21*(2), 145–152.

Rezansoff, S. N., Moniruzzaman, A., Clark, E., & Somers, J. M. (2015). Beyond recidivism: Changes in health and social service involvement following exposure to drug treatment court. *Substance Abuse Treatment, Prevention, and Policy, 10*, 42. doi:10.1186/s13011-015-0038-x.

Robert Wood Johnson Foundation (2014). *Evaluation of the Healthy Kids, Healthy Communities: Cross-site report*. Retrieved from: www.rwjf.org/en/library/research/2014/04/evaluation-of-healthy-kids--healthy-communities-cross-site-repor.html.

Rosenbaum, D. P., & Lawrence, D. S. (2011). Teaching respectful police-citizen encounters and good decision making: Results of a randomized control trial with police recruits. Washington, DC: National Police Research Platform.

Thornton, R. L. J., Greiner, A., Fichtenberg, C. M., Feingold, B. J., Ellen, J. M., & Jennings, J. M. (2013). Achieving a healthy zoning policy in Baltimore: Results of a health impact assessment of the Transform Baltimore zoning code rewrite. *Public Health Reports, 128*(6, Suppl. 3), 87–103.

Waddell, S. (1995). Lessons from the healthy cities movement for social indicator development. *Social Indicators Research, 34*(2), 213–235.

Wall, M., Hayes, R., Moore, D., Petticrew, M., Clow, A., Schmidt, E., … & Renton, A. (2009). Evaluation of community level interventions to address social and structural determinants of health: A cluster randomised controlled trial. *BMC Public Health, 9*, 207. doi:10.1186/1471-2458-9-207.

Wilkinson, R. G., & Marmot, M. (Eds.). (2003). *Social determinants of health: The solid facts*. World Health Organization. Retrieved from: https://books.google.com/books?hl=en&lr=&id=QDFzqNZZHLMC&oi=fnd&pg=PA5&dq=marmot+and+wilkinson+2003&ots=xVuJfBURju&sig=vgWIEX1gQapfhyZaHYcydGGFkCM#v=onepage&q=marmot%20and%20wilkinson%202003&f=false.

7 Case studies of a SDOH evaluation

Learning objectives

After reading this chapter, you should be able to:

- Be familiar with SDOH focused evaluation approaches and how to apply them to real-life evaluations
- Know how to determine data available that can be used in SDOH focused evaluations
- Describe methods used to develop SDOH evaluations
- Understand the role of funding agencies, programs, and policies as they view SDOH evaluations and their use

The names and data used in these case studies are made up and do not refer to any existing persons, programs, or situations.

For each of the case studies listed in this chapter we will review background information about the issue. Background information is useful for documenting the history of a program or why a specific evaluation is needed. Next, summary information about the program or team leading the effort is given. The following sections describe a process of determining which data is available for a SDOH evaluation. Remember, these are not real cases, so some of the SDOH indicators do not have actual values. Knowing what data is available and the methods that will be used in your evaluation is the next step. Next, a summary of an analysis plan and results are provided. Each case study moves forward two years in time. I realize this is somewhat unrealistic, but stay with me. The results from each of these case studies shed light on the findings and unique challenges that evaluators may experience as they implement SDOH evaluations. As you read these case studies, think about how they are similar to or different from evaluations that you may have conducted in the past. What is unique about the SDOH focus? At the same time, do you think it is possible that evaluators will experience resistance?

Jane was 40 when I met her. She was just beginning a degree program at the university I was working at. I recall meeting with her several times to discuss the program, prerequisites, and what to expect. I was impressed by her past experiences, her positive outlook on life, and her determination to better herself as the first person in her family to earn a college degree. Two weeks later I got the call. Jane passed away from complications related to drug and alcohol abuse. Jane would not start or finish the program. She would not meet her first grandchild or grow old with her family and friends. SDOH focused evaluations have the potential to change what we think we know about health, and what determines health in our world. Drug and alcohol abuse were not the cause of Jane's death, they were a symptom of conditions, position, vulnerability, and disadvantage.

Case study 1: State opioid SDOH evaluation

Background

The number of opioid-involved overdose deaths in the United States increased by 90% from 2013 to 2017 (Gladden, O'Donnell, Mattson, et al., 2019). One of the primary reasons for increases in overdose deaths is the combination of illicitly manufactured fentanyl mixed with heroin or mixed with counterfeit prescription pills. Opioid overdose deaths and the opioid crisis has devastating economic and societal impacts. In 2015, the US' estimated economic costs associated with the opioid crisis exceeded $504 billion, which was six times more than the original cost estimates (Council of Economic Advisers, 2017). Opioid-related fatality data from the CDC WONDER database shows that most deaths occur among individuals between the ages of 25 and 55 and the overall US fatality rate is 10.3 deaths per 100,000 population (CDC, 2019). Opioid-involved overdose deaths vary by state and region; during 2017, there were 2,199 overdose deaths involving opioids in California for a rate of 5.3 per 100,000 population (CDC, 2019).

Several factors may be linked to increases in opioid-involved overdose deaths. Opioid prescriptions for pain vary throughout the United States. In California, providers wrote 39.5 opioid prescriptions for everyone 100 persons, whereas, in contrast, the US rate for prescriptions was 58.7 per 100 (National Institute on Drug Abuse, 2018). Lower prescribing rates in California may result in fewer opioid-involved overdose deaths.

Public health officials predict that the opioid overdose crisis will worsen, and the annual number of opioid overdose deaths will reach nearly 82,000 by 2025; this would mean 700,000 deaths from 2016 to 2025 due to opioid overdose. Interventions that address the opioid crisis are projected to result in a 3% to 5% decrease in opioid overdose deaths (Chen, Larochelle, Weaver, et al., 2019). Prevention of prescription opioid misuse alone is not enough. A multipronged approach is needed to change the course of the epidemic; this approach would include addressing the SDOH.

This background sets the stage for a SDOH focused evaluation in the State of California. Building on previous chapters and content outlined throughout this text, this case study outlines a process for conducting a SDOH focused evaluation.

Program

The State of California received funding from the Substance Abuse and Mental Health Services Administration (SAMHSA) to develop a program that would address the opioid crisis by reducing unmet treatment need and reducing opioid overdose–related deaths through the provision of prevention, treatment, and recovery activities for opioid use disorder (OUD). The primary goals of the evaluation were to target intervention points while changing the social and economic structure of communities that unfairly serves males, African Americans, Native Americans, and individuals with lower social capital. These populations were selected because they are placed at higher risk for OUD.

Establish a team

The California State Health Department asked local public health officials to convene a diverse team of public health professionals familiar with the opioid crisis to help develop a SDOH focused evaluation. State officials wanted to know the underlying causes of opioid use and opioid-involved deaths. Funding from SAMHSA allowed the public health agencies to implement a variety of activities to address treatment needs, prevention, and recovery services.

The team met on November 1, 2019. They were selected by state, local, county, and tribal officials for their experience and knowledge. Some had the lived experience of addiction or past opioid use, while others were impacted more indirectly, by family, friends, neighbors, or clinical environments where demands from the opioid crisis were increasing. During the first meeting, team members introduced themselves and why they wanted to attend the meeting. After brief introductions, the Project Director developed a list of competencies and skills that members of the team possessed, and these are summarized below:

- Experience with public health evaluation and OUD
- Knowledge of opioid-involved mortality risk and protective factors
- Awareness of current state policies, procedures, programs, and initiatives to address the opioid crisis
- Knowledge of medication assisted treatment, prevention, and recovery services
- Experience with systems thinking and the socioecological model in evaluation

Team members spent time discussing their capacities and what made them uniquely qualified to assist with the SDOH focused evaluation. A list of potential contributions from various team members was compiled to identify knowledge and service gaps for the SDOH focused evaluation, and this is set out in Table 7.1.

Table 7.1 Team members and contributions

Team Members	Potential Contributions to Evaluation
Project Director	Manage project, budgets, timeline, long-term programming
Evaluator	Plan and design evaluation, identify existing data, link determinants, implement evaluation, analyze data and report results
Community partners, individuals with lived experience of opioid use	Assist with design, interpreting results, reporting results back, education
State, local, and community-based organizations	Assist with design, reporting, policy change, housing, workforce development
Clinical staff	Assist with education about OUD, reporting, clinical care/treatment, policy and systems change

Determine data available

After the evaluator and clinical staff conducted a literature review on the opioid crisis and potential SDOH determinants, the team met to discuss these and develop a conceptual framework for designing the evaluation. This process was participatory and collaborative, engaging professionals, the state, and individuals with the lived experience of being impacted by the opioid crisis during the process.

SDOH team members focused their SDOH evaluation to explore the following:

- What are the evidence-based determinants of opioid-involved deaths?
- What are other determinants identified by the community or geographic location?
- How will the program address these determinants?
- How long will this take?
- How much will this program cost?
- What resources are needed?
- How will you know if you have accomplished your goals in addressing the social determinants?

The team used the initiative planning model discussed in Chapter 3 to create a plan that would include SDOH in the program evaluation approach. This is illustrated in Figure 7.1.

To increase understanding about SDOH and an evaluation that utilizes the SDOH, team members completed a six-hour training facilitated by the evaluator and clinical team member. This training was informed by existing literature on SDOH and what is known about SDOH and opioid-involved overdose deaths. Team members learned how to conduct interviews, record data, and report information back to the larger group while maintaining confidentiality. The opioid program was successfully implemented over a two-year period.

Goal: To improve social determinants in order to reduce opioid involved deaths

Guiding Questions	Individual Objective:	Organizational Objective:	Community Objective:
What are the evidence-based determinants?	By 2020, increase awareness of social determinants of OUD and opioid-involved deaths	By 2021, increase the number and reach of opioid prevention programs that help target population	By 2022, increase number of individuals in permanent housing
What other determinants are identified by the community?	**Approach:** Consciousness raising	**Approach:** Program development	**Approach:** Policy change
What will you do?	**Action Steps:** Create media campaign that educates policy makers, families, law enforcement, schools, and community members	**Action Steps:** Work with existing programs, policy leaders, and funders to expand prevention programming and address racial disadvantage	**Action Steps:** Work with state, federal officials to change housing eviction policies
How long will it take? How much does it cost?			
What resources are needed?			**Resources & Costs:** Staff, grant funding or 3rd party billing for prevention, facilities, outreach efforts
How will you know if you have accomplished your goal?	**Resources & Costs:** Staff, media materials, billboard fees, web designer	**Resources & Costs:** Staff, Medicaid, grant funding or 3rd party billing for prevention, facilities, outreach efforts	

Figure 7.1 Initiative planning model to reduce opioid-involved deaths.

Identify appropriate methods

After reviewing data available the team decided to frame the evaluation using the health equity conceptual framework summarized in Chapter 3. Figure 7.2 demonstrates an application of this framework to the present evaluation around the opioid crisis and current program funding to address unmet needs.

Team members agreed they would use both qualitative and quantitative data in the evaluation—this resulted in a mixed-method evaluation approach, where qualitative data could help inform questions about SDOH that quantitative data could not. Team members at the State of California were familiar with existing OUD data and recommended utilizing this data in addition to the Social Needs Screening Tool.

Participants receiving services from the program would complete this tool at intake, at 90 days, at six months, and at discharge. Domains include race or ethnic group, education, financial strain, stress, depression, physical activity, opioid use, alcohol and other drug use, social connections or isolation, intimate partner violence, and median income. The team added housing status and involvement in workforce development programs to the questionnaire to capture SDOH intervention points outlined in Figure 7.1. The domains are shown in Table 7.2.

Qualitative data would be collected using semi-structured interviews with individuals with the lived experience of OUD, family members, and clinical team members. An interview guide was developed by the team and piloted prior to data collection; it was tested with representative members of the population

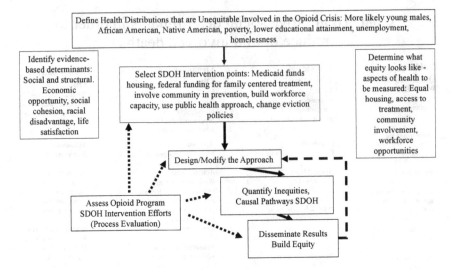

Figure 7.2 Health equity evaluation for opioid crisis.

Source: Adapted from Dover & Belon (2019).

Table 7.2 Social and behavioral domains and measures to address the opioid crisis

Domain	Measure	Change Rate
Race or Ethnic Group	Race, Hispanic, Latino, or Spanish origin	At intake
Education	Highest level school completed; highest degree earned	At intake
Financial Strain	Difficulty paying for food, housing, medical care, heat	At intake, follow-up
Stress	Feeling restless, nervous, anxious, unable to sleep	At intake, follow-up
Depression	Past two weeks little interests in pleasure, feeling down, depressed, hopeless	At intake, follow-up
Physical Activity	Days per week moderate exercise, minutes engaged	At intake, follow-up
Tobacco Use	Lifetime cigarette use, current cigarette/tobacco use	At intake, follow-up
Alcohol Use	Frequency of alcohol intake, daily intake, binge drinking	At intake, follow-up
Other Drug Use	Frequency of drug use, intake, daily intake, binge drinking	At intake, follow-up
Opioid Use	Frequency of opioid, intake, daily intake, binge drinking	At intake, follow-up
Social Connections or Isolation	Frequency of talking and gathering with friends, attending church services, attending meetings or organizations	At intake, follow-up

Domain	Measure	Change Rate
Intimate Partner Violence	Past year humiliated or emotionally abused by partner/ex-partner, afraid, physically hurt	At intake, follow-up
Monthly Income	Current monthly income	At intake, follow-up
Housing Status	Current housing status	At intake, follow-up
Workforce Development	Current participation in workforce development, skill building programs	At intake, follow-up
Recovery and Treatment	Current participation in recovery and treatment activities	At intake, follow-up
Workforce Development	Current participation in workforce development, skill building programs	At intake, follow-up

Source: Adapted from Adler & Stead (2015).

that would be interviewed. A consent form outlined the purpose of the interviews, how information would be used, and potential risks associated with the interviews. Copies of consent forms were given to individuals interviewed for recordkeeping purposes. For completing the social needs screening survey and interviews, individuals were compensated with a $25 gift card.

Results

The program implemented a multipronged approach that increased prevention strategies, access to treatment and recovery, and response to opioid-involved overdoses. Prevention strategies included safer prescribing and dispensing, education and stigma reduction, and monitoring and communication. Education focused on harm reduction, community dialogue about non-stigmatizing language to change perceptions about OUD, and community-based medication disposal programs, drop boxes, and participation in national prescription take back days. Treatment and recovery program activities increased access to care through Medicaid funding and funding for family treatment approaches. Recovery support activities also increased workforce capacity and skills as well as access to sober activities in the communities. Program response efforts included training individuals to administer naloxone in the event of an overdose and changing eviction policies for individuals who have criminal records for opioid-related crimes and use. At the policy level, the program was involved in federal addiction legislation such as the 2016 Comprehensive Addiction Recovery Act.

Two years later

The program ended and the evaluation reports document the process and impact of the program on addressing the opioid crisis using the SDOH. Program staff knew what the evidence-based determinants of opioid-involved deaths were, based on previous literature. These were social and structural in nature, including economic opportunity, social cohesion, racial disadvantage, and life satisfaction. Other determinants identified by the community were the need to support housing with Medicaid funding and changing eviction policies for individuals with opioid use disorder. The program implemented a variety of services throughout the state to intervene and reduce opioid-involved deaths while increasing access to medication assisted treatment, prevention, and recovery support services.

Policy change to address Medicaid funding and eviction notices was just emerging at the end of the grant, gaining momentum and with bills before the legislature that would provide greater housing support for individuals in need. This demonstrates that when addressing the SDOH using a population health approach, it may take longer to document actualized results than with non-SDOH focused interventions. At the agency level, more providers are utilizing evidence-based treatment and people qualified to prescribe medication assisted treatment. These two outcomes are directly linked to the program efforts. Resources needed to implement the program were enough, yet the sustainability of the program efforts is a major concern. With limited funding, additional programming to address the opioid crisis will be difficult to implement.

Case study 2: Evaluation of SDOH and substance use and mental health

Background

Substance use and poor mental health conditions (SUMH) together have given rise to one of the most pressing public health emergencies of the century. Since 1990, SUMH conditions have increased 38% in the world (Whiteford, Degenhardt, Rehm, et al., 2013). The US has witnessed similar increases in SUMH conditions. Despite public health and policy efforts to reduce substance use (SU), rates have remained the same since 2002—binge drinking (23%) and illicit drug use (8.3%) (Center for Behavioral Health Statistics and Quality, 2015). Mental health disorders are one of the top five causes of disability in the US.

Some populations may be more vulnerable to SUMH conditions than others. Racial/ethnic populations may be placed at greater risk due to trauma, discrimination, socioeconomic conditions, and structural inequalities that fail to support health equity.

The purpose of this evaluation was to examine the SDOH as they relate to SUMH in Oregon and Washington. This evaluation focused on SDOH that have been identified in the literature: race/ethnic group, income/unemployment, poverty, education, violent crime, severe housing, percentage rural, and percentage uninsured. The primary question this study seeks to answer is: "Are there differences in SDOH that could explain SUMH disparities in Oregon and Washington?"

Program

The Healthy Communities program was led by a community-based consortium in downtown Seattle, Washington. The program has a long history of providing mental health and SU services for vulnerable populations in the Oregon and Washington areas. With new funding from a private foundation, the team explored the SDOH of SUMH to understand more about the structural factors that may contribute to inequalities in health among populations served by the Healthy Communities program. Conducting a literature review and exploring existing data available was a first step in the Healthy Communities program project. Information that resulted from this effort will be used by the team to develop a SDOH focused intervention and subsequent evaluation.

Establish a team

The Healthy Communities 10-member team included consortium staff, state, local, and county officials, community members, and clinicians. Some had the lived experience of SU disorder and poor mental health, while others were impacted more indirectly, by family, friends, neighbors, or clinical environments where demands for effective treatment were increasing. After brief introductions, the Project Director developed a list of competencies and skills that members of the team possessed, and these are summarized below:

- Experience with public health evaluation and SUMH
- Knowledge of risk and protective factors associated with SDOH and SUMH
- Awareness of current state policies, procedures, programs, and initiatives to address SDOH and SUMH
- Knowledge of treatment, prevention, and recovery services
- Experience with systems thinking and the socioecological model in evaluation

Values guiding healthy communities

Team members spent time discussing their capacities and what made them uniquely qualified to assist with the SDOH literature review and eventually a SDOH focused evaluation.

Healthy Communities utilized the CIRCLE (Community Involvement to Renew Commitment, Leadership, and Effectiveness) model which parallels a Community-Based Participatory Research (CBPR) approach and focuses on building relationships, building skills, working together, and promoting commitment (Chino, Dodge-Francis, DeBruyn, et al., 2012). Importantly, this model prompts healthier communities and supports moving away from risk factors associated with SUMH by promoting change in the risk conditions that contribute to health disparities. Shifting from a traditional CBPR approach to a CIRCLE approach led to more successful community-based interventions. The first step of creating the CIRCLE was to promote the concept of "belonging," whereby community members, staff, team members, and partners felt comfortable sharing information and their presence was acknowledged by others as important. Second, Healthy Communities provided skill building opportunities based on community identified needs. An example of this was practicing empowerment evaluation principles and group facilitation strategies. The third step required the community members to work collaboratively together, also referred to as interdependence. This acknowledged that community members are inextricably linked to their family, culture, and environment. The last step of the CIRCLE was to promote commitment; this is also referred to as generosity, whereby respected members of the consortium and community provide knowledge and give back to the community. This was incorporated into the last phase of the study and future interventions.

Determine data available

After the evaluator and consortium staff conducted a literature review on SUMH and SDOH, the team met to discuss these and develop a conceptual framework for designing the evaluation. This process was participatory and collaborative, engaging professionals, the state, and individuals with the lived experience of SUMH.

SDOH team members focused their SDOH evaluation to explore several important questions. The first three questions were answered during the literature review process and review/analysis of existing data.

- What are the evidence-based determinants of SUMH?
- What are other determinants identified by the community or geographic location?
- How will the program address these determinants?
- How long will this take?
- How much will this program cost?
- What resources are needed?
- How will you know if you have accomplished your goals in addressing the social determinants?

Identify appropriate methods

The team selected a cross-sectional study design to explore SDOH and SUMH in 79 counties in Oregon and Washington. This evaluation was guided by the question, "Are there differences in SDOH that could explain SUMH disparities in racial/ethnic populations in Oregon and Washington counties?"

Data sources and variables

Publicly available data from multiple databases was used to examine the SDOH and SUMH by county.

Table 7.3 summarizes data sources and variables used.

Table 7.3 Data sources, variables, and SDOH pathways

Data Source	Variables	SDOH Pathway
Economic Research Service	Unemployment, poverty, and high school diploma	Socioeconomic conditions Political conditions
Robert Wood Johnson Foundation County Health Rankings	Excessive drinking, poor mental health, percent rural	Health behaviors and circumstances Rural and limited access to services/isolation
Comprehensive Housing Affordability Strategy	Severe housing problems	Environment
Federal Bureau of Investigations Uniform Crime Reporting	Violent crime	Environment Institutional Political
Centers for Disease Control WONDER Mortality Data	Drug poisoning death	Health care and treatment access Health behaviors
US Census Population Estimates from the American Community Survey	Percent racial/ethnic minority and non-Hispanic White	Community conditions Vulnerable populations

Independent variables. Unemployment, poverty all ages, no high school diploma, percentage rural, percentage uninsured, percentage racial ethnic minority, violent crime rate, and severe housing problems were the independent SDOH variables.

Dependent variable. The dependent variable, SUMH, was created by combining the number of excessive drinking days in the past 30 days and the number of poor mental health days in the past 30 days for each county. Drug poisoning deaths were explored as a variable but not included due to the large number of missing cases.

Figure 7.3 highlights the SDOH and potential targets for intervention to reduce differences in SUMH and SDOH experienced by racial/ethnic minorities.

Results

Descriptive statistics were used to examine all variables of interest. Table 7.4 shows mean scores for each SDOH characteristic by state and rural designation. Mean and percentage scores of unemployment, poverty, no high school diploma, excessive drinking, violent crime rate, severe housing problems, rural location, and uninsured adults were higher in rural areas compared with all Oregon and Washington counties. Poor mental health days and drug poisoning deaths were higher in non-CHSDA (contract health service delivery area) counties.

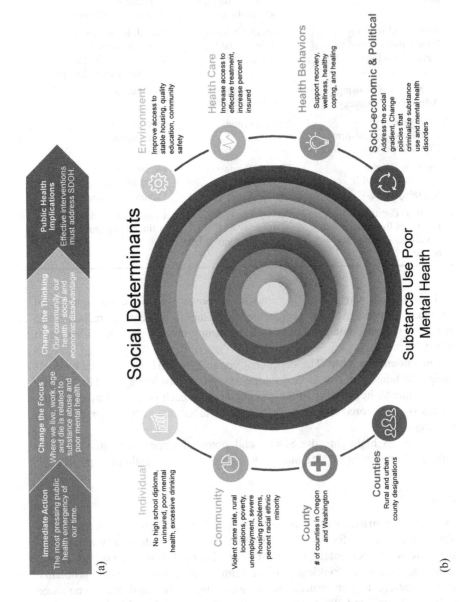

(a)

Immediate Action
The most pressing public health emergency of our time.

Change the Focus
Where we live, work, age and die is related to substance abuse and poor mental health.

Change the Thinking
Our community, our health - social and economic disadvantage.

Public Health Implications
Effective interventions must address SDOH.

Social Determinants

Environment
Improve access to stable housing, quality education, community safety

Health Care
Increase access to effective treatment, increase percent insured

Health Behaviors
Support recovery, wellness, healthy coping, and healing

Socio-economic & Political
Address the social gradient. Change policies that criminalize substance use and mental health disorders

Individual
No high school diploma, uninsured, poor mental health, excessive drinking

Community
Violent crime rate, rural locations, poverty, unemployment, severe housing problems, percent racial ethnic minority

County
# of counties in Oregon and Washington

Counties
Rural and urban county designations

Substance Use Poor Mental Health

(b)

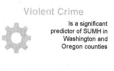

Violent Crime

Is a significant
predictor of SUMH in
Washington and
Oregon counties

Drug Poisoning Deaths

Positively associated
with no high school
diploma in Washington
and Oregon counties

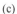

Poverty

Is an underlying
factor contributing
to substance abuse
and poor mental
health in Washington
and Oregon counties

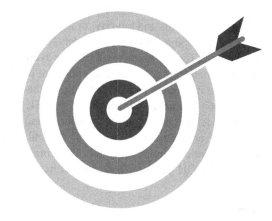

(c)

Figure 7.3 Conceptualizing social determinants of substance use and poor mental health.

Note

In Figure 7.3b, the individual level is at the center of the circle, and the socioeconomic/political level is represented by the outer circle, with the other levels arranged between them.

Table 7.4 Comparison of counties and SDOH characteristics

SDOH Characteristics	Oregon (RWJF, 2019a)	Washington (RWJF, 2019b)	US	Rural
Characteristic Mean or %SD				
Unemployment %	4.1%	4.8%	4.4%	*
Percent Children Poverty	17%	14%	18%	*
Percent 9th Graders Graduating in Four Years	77%	79%	85%	*
Percent Excessive Drinking Past 30 days	19%	18%	18%	*
Number of Poor Mental Health Days Past 30 days	4.5	3.8	3.8	*
Violent Crime Rate per 100,000 population	249	294	286	*
Percent Households with Overcrowding, High Costs, Lack of Plumbing	20%	28%	33%	*
Drug Poisoning Deaths per 100,000 population	*	*	*	*
Percent Under Age 65 Uninsured	7%	7%	10%	*
Percent Rural	30.5%	31.1%	19.3% (US Census, 2016)	*

Note

*Data not included in this table because it was not available, and this is a case example.

Results suggest that relationships between SDOH variables were statistically significant. The strongest correlations were observed for the following SDOH: racial ethnic minority status and poverty, drug poisoning deaths and poor mental health, and drug poisoning deaths and no high school diploma. Inverse relationships were observed for the following SDOH: poverty and non-Hispanic White, uninsured and non-Hispanic White. One important observation from this correlation matrix is the difference in SDOH based on the percentage of racial/ethnic minorities and non-Hispanic Whites. Most SDOH were positively correlated with percentage racial/ethnic minority by county and negatively correlated with the percentage of non-Hispanic Whites. In general, these results suggest that racial/ethnic populations in Oregon and Washington may experience greater vulnerabilities to SDOH than non-Hispanic Whites.

Implications

The implications of this evaluation are numerous. First, prevention and treatment of SUMH is costly and, without insurance, many people do not have access to the services they need. Second, counties with a higher percentage of racial/ethnic minorities and rural status experience greater SUMH needs due to the social and economic factors that shape health and behaviors. This is consistent with previous literature, in which communities impacted by political, economic, and social disadvantage have been shown more likely to experience health inequalities (Whitehead & Dahlgren, 2006). Third, this study found a significant association between SDOH and SUMH in Oregon and Washington—these findings must be used to inform future policy, prevention, and intervention efforts that utilize the SDOH framework. Fourth, all SDOH were positively correlated with percentage racial/ethnic minority, indicating that these populations are placed at greater risk for SUMH than non-Hispanic Whites in Oregon and Washington counties. Fifth, poverty was the strongest predictor of SUMH, followed by no high school diploma. The implications of these findings combined are that interventions must address the social gradient, support vulnerable populations, improve living conditions, and reduce risk conditions to promote health equity.

Two years later

The Healthy Communities program used information from the literature review and secondary data analysis to develop a SDOH focused intervention for areas served by the Healthy Communities Program SU and mental health programs. The SDOH intervention utilized the Medicaid 1115 waiver program to improve services for clients so that they would be holistic and support mental well-being and recovery. At the end of the program, 100 clients received expanded services, peer recovery support, work force development preparation, education and GED support, and resources that would improve housing access and quality in rural areas. The team felt that two years was not a sufficient amount of time to implement the SDOH intervention, and evaluation results did not tell the entire story of the profound impact the intervention had on individuals, families, and communities. Healthy Communities plans to continue its work and seek additional funding and support for SDOH focused interventions.

Case study 3: Type 2 diabetes and SDOH

Background

Diabetes is a public health epidemic. Type 2 diabetes (T2D) is preventable yet rates continue to climb and by 2050, one in three adults could have diabetes (CDC, 2011). Data from the 1995, 2000, 2005, and 2010 Behavioral Risk Factor Surveillance System (BRFSS) shows consistent and alarming increases in diabetes prevalence, ranging from 8.5% to more than 225% in some states (CDC, 2013). Individuals living in rural areas experience higher rates of diabetes than those living in urban areas. Racial and ethnic minorities are disproportionately impacted by diabetes, and among certain populations throughout the US, diabetes prevalence continues to increase. Efforts to address diabetes have focused on the etiology, biology, and prevalence of diabetes in segments of a given population, and on health care delivery standards. Often these efforts focus on lifestyle and behavior modification grounded in various individual theories such as social cognitive theory or the health belief model. Theories and efforts have led to numerous initiatives to increase physical activity and promote healthy eating. However, most initiatives have not been successful in reducing the incidence of diabetes at the individual or population level. Initiatives rarely address the underlying reasons for diabetes—namely, the social and environmental conditions, or SDOH, that influence the modifiable risk factors. The SDOH framework is emerging as a key conceptual tool for understanding the causes of diabetes and potential solutions to reverse the diabetes epidemic, especially among vulnerable populations (Marmot, 2005).

Only a limited number of studies have applied the SDOH framework to population-level characteristics with the aim of better understanding the risk conditions associated with diabetes. Therefore, the purpose of this study was to determine if indicators of the SDOH are useful predictors of diabetes prevalence in the United States. The SDOH in this evaluation were selected based on the Healthy People 2020 SDOH framework and categorized based on education, economic stability, neighborhood and built environment, health and health care, and social and community context.

Establish a team

A local university received funding to explore SDOH and diabetes prevalence. The university asked local public health officials, state, local, and county officials, and community members to serve as a community advisory board for the project. During the first meeting, team members introduced themselves and why they wanted to attend the meeting. After brief introductions, the university evaluator developed a list of competencies and skills that members of the team possessed, and these are summarized below:

- Experience with public health evaluation
- Knowledge of T2D risk and protective factors
- Awareness of current state policies, procedures, programs, and initiatives to address T2D

Team members spent time discussing their capacities and what made them uniquely qualified to assist with the SDOH focused evaluation. After this initial meeting, team members decided on potential roles, and used the four-step SDOH evaluation framework presented earlier in this text to plan the evaluation.

Determine data available

After completing a literature review on potential SDOH, the team met to discuss it and develop a conceptual framework for designing the evaluation. This process was participatory and collaborative, engaging both clinical and community members in the process.

SDOH team members focused their SDOH evaluation to explore the following:

- What are the evidence-based determinants of T2D?
- What are other determinants identified by the community or geographic location?
- What kinds of programs are needed to address these determinants?
- How long will this take?
- How much will this program cost?
- What resources are needed?
- How will you know if you have accomplished your goals in addressing the social determinants?

Identify appropriate methods

After reviewing data available the team decided to frame the evaluation using the health impact pyramid to illustrate the levels in which interventions could have the greatest impact. The base level of the pyramid includes the socioeconomic determinants of T2D from the literature, then public health interventions that change conditions for health, protective interventions that have long-term impact, clinical care, and counseling and education. This was an appropriate framework because the team was interested in developing interventions and programming that would target the pyramid base (socioeconomic determinants). A cross-sectional ecological study design was used to compare diabetes prevalence by county in the US. The SDOH approach was warranted because previous literature in other populations had shown that certain SDOH were associated with health disparities in T2D. Team members agreed they would use only quantitative data in the evaluation.

Publicly available data from multiple databases was used to examine the SDOH and diabetes prevalence by county. Diabetes prevalence, obesity, smoking, and physical inactivity data was extracted from the 2014 BRFSS based on county level estimates (www.cdc.gov/brfss/index.html). BRFSS is a national random digit dial telephone survey representative of the total non-institutionalized population over 18 years of age living in households with a land line telephone. Data from the 2014 ACS (www.census.gov/programs-surveys/acs/) was used to document the percentage of persons with college degrees and percentage racial/ ethnic populations. Data from the 2014 Economic Research Service (ERS, www.ers.usda.gov/) was used to designate counties with housing stress, low education, low employment, persistent poverty, and persistent child poverty. Data from the USDA Food Environment Atlas 2014 (www.ers.usda.gov/ foodatlas/) was used to assess the percentage of county population with limited food access.

Data was analyzed using descriptive statistics, and a correlation matrix was created for all variables with the outcome of diabetes prevalence. Multiple regression analyses were used to assess the most useful SDOH predictors of diabetes prevalence in preliminary models.

Results

Results from the data analyses show variance in diabetes prevalence throughout the US. All SDOH predictor variables were associated with SDOH and this was expected. SDOH were useful in predicting diabetes prevalence, with college degree and rural locations being the strongest predictors. Limited food access was also a significant predictor of diabetes prevalence in the sample.

The university team used the results to develop a statewide program to target SDOH identified in this study. Program strategies included college readiness, and high school graduation and testing preparation support. Team members identified rural locations in their state and potential partners and policies that would bring additional resources into these areas, including increasing healthy food access.

Two years later

Team members celebrate the widely successfully SDOH program that reduced diabetes prevalence in their state. Results from the evaluation indicate that high school graduation rates have improved, and that resources expended on testing and college prep have increased access to college degrees. Community gardens and healthy food retail interventions have increased healthy food access in rural and urban locations throughout the state. Although it will take time to see the full impact of this program, the team is hopeful that college graduation rates will improve, and diabetes prevalence will continue to decrease.

Summary of case studies

These case examples demonstrates how evaluations can address the underlying conditions of a public health problem, more than just looking at a single health outcome, and how, in these cases, opioid-involved overdose deaths, opioid use, SU and poor mental health, or T2D prevalence are influenced by SDOH. In some cases, funding agencies supporting these programs did not require a SDOH focused evaluation, but teams felt it was important to address because substance misuse and abuse, poor mental health, opioid-involved overdose deaths, and T2D are not distributed equally among the US population. Using existing studies, existing literature, and a team approach, these case examples identify the populations that were placed at highest risk, the evidence-based determinants, potential intervention points, and processes to measure interventions throughout the two-year program. What seems to be clear from these case studies is that the SDOH framework can change population-level risk conditions that lead to poorer health outcomes. Ultimately, findings from these studies have the potential to increase understanding about the associations of SDOH and evaluation in the US and beyond.

Points to remember

1   Just because a program does not have a SDOH focus does not mean that the evaluation should not have one. In these examples, teams collected additional data from participants that captured SDOH areas identified in the initiative planning model and health equity model. Teams also reviewed SDOH data using secondary data sources, as this was more efficient and less costly to the program.

2   Use the models presented throughout this text as a guide—there are even more available, and sometimes more than one may be appropriate. For example, the socioecological model could easily have been used to explore the SDOH related to the opioid crisis and intervention points based on individual or policy realms.

3   Evaluating the SDOH takes time, and policy change will not occur overnight. I encourage evaluators to look back, in one year, five years, or 10 years to see what the impact was of a program on a desired health outcome, especially those that determine our health.

4   Having a team to assist with education about SDOH, discussing approaches to evaluating programs using the SDOH focus, and disseminating results is critical.

References

Adler, N. E., & Stead, W. W. (2015). Patients in context: EHR capture of social and behavioral determinants of health. *New England Journal of Medicine, 372*(8), 698–701.

Center for Behavioral Health Statistics and Quality. (2015). Behavioral health trends in the United States: Results from the 2014 National Survey on Drug Use and Health.

Rockville, MD: Substance Abuse and Mental Health Services Administration (HHS Publication No SMA 15-4927 NSDUH Series H-5).

Centers for Disease Control and Prevention. (2011). National diabetes fact sheet: National estimates and general information on diabetes and prediabetes in the United States. Atlanta, GA: CDC.

Centers for Disease Control and Prevention. (2013). Behavioral risk factor surveillance system: Diabetes, obesity, physical inactivity by state and county, 2004. Retrieved from: www.cdc.gov/brfss/annual_data/annual_2004.htm.

Centers for Disease Control and Prevention. (2019). Multiple cause of death data. Retrieved from: https://wonder.cdc.gov/.

Chen, Q., Larochelle, M. R., Weaver, D. T., Lietz, A. P., Mueller, P. P., Mercaldo, S., ... & Chhatwal, J. (2019). Prevention of prescription opioid misuse and projected overdose deaths in the United States. *JAMA* network open, *2*(2), e187621. doi:10.1001/jamanetworkopen.2018.7621.

Chino, M., Dodge-Francis, C., DeBruyn, L., Short, L., & Satterfield, D. (2012). The convergence of science and culture: Developing a framework for diabetes education in tribal communities. *Journal of Health Disparities Research and Practice, 1*(3): 7.

Council of Economic Advisers (2017, November). The underestimated costs of the opioid crisis. White House. Retrieved from: www.whitehouse.gov/sites/whitehouse.gov/files/images/The%20Underestimated%20Cost%20of%20the%20Opioid%20Crisis.pdf.

Dover, D., & Belon, A. (2019). The health equity measurement framework: A comprehensive model to measure social inequities in health. *International Journal for Equity in Health, 18*(1), 36. doi:10.1186/s12939-019-0935-0.

Gladden, R., O'Donnell, J., Mattson, C., & Seth, P. (2019). Changes in opioid-involved overdose deaths by opioid type and presence of benzodiazepines, cocaine, and methamphetamine: 25 states, July–December 2017 to January–June 2018. *MMWR Morbidity and Mortality Weekly Report, 68*(34), 737–744. doi:10.15585/mmwr.mm6834a2externalicon.

Marmot, M. (2005). Social determinants of health inequalities. *The Lancet, 365*(9464), 1099–1104.

National Institute on Drug Abuse. (2018). Opioid involved overdose deaths by state. California. Retrieved from: www.drugabuse.gov/drugs-abuse/opioids/opioid-summaries-by-state/california-opioid-summary.

Robert Wood Johnson Foundation. (2019a). County health rankings for Oregon measures and national/state results. Available from: www.countyhealthrankings.org/reports/state-reports/2019-oregon-report.

Robert Wood Johnson Foundation. (2019b). County health rankings for Washington measures and national/state results. Available from: www.countyhealthrankings.org/reports/state-reports/2019-washington-report.

US Census (2016). New census data show differences between urban and rural populations. Available from: www.census.gov/newsroom/press-releases/2016/cb16-210.html.

Whiteford, H. A., Degenhardt, L., Rehm, J., Baxter, A. J., Ferrari, A. J., Erskine, H. E., ... & Burstein, R. (2013). Global burden of disease attributable to mental and substance use disorders: Findings from the Global Burden of Disease Study 2010. *The Lancet, 382*(9904), 1575–1586.

Whitehead, M., & Dahlgren, G. (2006). Concepts and principles for tackling social inequities in health: Levelling up Part 1. Studies on social and economic determinants of population health, No. 2. Copenhagen, Denmark: World Health Organization.

8   Bringing it all together

Learning objectives

After reading this chapter, you should be able to:

*   Summarize SDOH
*   Describe SDOH evaluation approaches
*   Summarize SDOH challenges
*   List SDOH solutions
*   Describe differences in SDOH
*   Articulate plans for how to move forward with SDOH evaluation

Summary of SDOH

Public health as a discipline and way of life has come a long way since 1854 when John Snow identified the source of a cholera outbreak and prevented the deaths of thousands of people. He knew the source of the exposure (cause) and the impact (effect) it had on the health of the population. In this text we have explored the SDOH through different approaches, paradigms, programs, and thinking. Although the focus on SDOH has been in place since 1946 when the constitution of WHO was first drafted, there is still work that needs to be done. This constitution was developed to address the social roots of health problems globally, and to address challenges related to medical care delivery. Their goal was that all people would attain the highest possible level of mental, physical, and social well-being.

Isaac started smoking at the age of 10. The year was 1929 and the evidence demonstrating that smoking was bad for your health was not available. Isaac smoked throughout this childhood, as a member of the US Army in World War II, and then as an auto parts mechanic. He did not die from lung cancer, but smoking impacted his quality of life.

Moving forward 100 years, we have the evidence, smoking is not good for your health, but people continue to smoke. We do not have enough evidence about the social causes of disease, but we are making progress. I believe that in 100 years, the social causes of disease will be just as clear as the evidence base for smoking and lung cancer. This is why SDOH and public health evaluation matter.

Over time, as described in previous chapters, new public policies have been made, such as those cited in the Lalonde report that encouraged governments to recognize the importance of upstream policy agendas. Later, the Alma Ata Declaration was developed by world health leaders and linked primary health care to health inequalities. Later, in 1982, the *Black Report* documented inequalities in health based on social conditions. Work at WHO continued with the Health for All Approach, and the Ottawa Charter, designed to reduce health inequalities through social justice. Efforts in London and the US followed, with various initiatives designed to improve research and policy interventions that would address health inequalities. Research soon caught up with policies and declarations when the IOM report found that the US was failing in areas of population health, and that human potential, relationships, and political participation were necessary. Moving forward, Wilkinson and Marmot's work on the 10 solid SDOH facts linked socioeconomic conditions and health behaviors to poor health outcomes and urged the world to change how it thought about health equity and health disparities. Then, in 2008, the WHO Commission called for more action and made three recommendations grounded in SDOH (improve daily conditions, tackle inequity, and measure, understand, and assess the impact of actions). Shortly after this, the Rio Political Declaration on SDOH was adopted by 120 member states and this event created nine knowledge networks to improve SDOH action areas and prompt change. In the US, continued efforts like Healthy People 2020 and the Health Impact in 5 Years initiative seek to build community-wide approaches that promote positive health.

One of the observations that you might have after reading and knowing this history is that change takes time. Leaders, advocates, visionaries, experts, and communities have come together for more than half of a decade and called for action to address SDOH. These agreements have been slow to take hold or shift policy and funding toward an upstream approach. As we near the end of this text, we must think critically about our next steps. Where are we at and where do we need to go with SDOH focused programs and evaluations in public health?

SDOH evaluation

In this text we explored some evaluation approaches and program examples for conducting SDOH evaluations. We focused on the use of process and outcome evaluation in the design of SDOH focused efforts, but there are many more approaches that you should become familiar with. Other SDOH evaluation approaches that may be appropriate include: objectives oriented evaluation, expertise oriented evaluation, participant oriented evaluation, participatory and collaborative evaluation, cluster evaluation, evaluability assessment, objectives based evaluation, empowerment evaluation, participatory rural appraisal, utilization focused evaluation, theory driven evaluation, informal and formal evaluation, performance monitoring, impact evaluation, economic evaluation, and several others. Because there are libraries filled with textbooks on these evaluation approaches we did not explore the details of each.

Selecting an evaluation approach is not where the process ends. There are questions that we need to ask ourselves when approaching an evaluation that will include a SDOH component.

- What are the purposes of SDOH evaluation?
- What aspects of public health programs and SDOH should be evaluated?
- Who wants the evaluation and why?
- Who is doing the evaluation and what do they know about SDOH and community conditions that promote or take away from health?

We cannot answer these questions alone, but we must look to community members, leaders, advocates, professionals, and those who will be impacted by the evaluation first. This process of engaging others is critical in the development of a SDOH evaluation.

Once these questions are answered, one remains. How should the evaluation be conducted? In this text we proposed a four-step evaluation process. This process starts with **Step 1**, select a SDOH. This step involves reviewing literature on the specific determinant or health outcome and then developing goals that will support this area of inquiry. **Step 2** is about knowing when to use SDOH focused evaluations, and when to save them for a later time. You might think that all health outcomes have a social or economic cause, and while many social scientists would agree, there are some instances when SDOH focused evaluations are not appropriate. In Chapter 3 we discussed some of these—the biggest thing to know is this, do not use a SDOH focused evaluation if there is no support for or interest in exploring, understanding, or changing SDOH pathways or structural determinants that contribute to health inequities. Do use SDOH focused evaluations when you are evaluating policies, laws, community conditions, social conditions, socioeconomic conditions, culture, transportation, and the list goes on. I do not want to deter you from SDOH focused evaluations, but they do take time and sometimes this time is more than you have in a program evaluation time period. The costs and focus on outcomes that may not be related to the program goals or objectives can also be a sign that a SDOH focused evaluation is not appropriate. **Step 3** in the SDOH evaluation process is selecting a theory and knowing paradigms and frameworks. There are multiple theories that could be used to explore SDOH and inform evaluation planning and implementations. Although we will not go in detail, one important theory that underpins most evaluations is the theory of change. Theory of change describes what you think will happen as a result of a program or intervention and why this will happen. Appendix B has examples of theory of change models from previous SDOH evaluations. There are other theories too, and you may use multiple theories in your work. Paradigms are another area that evaluators must be aware of because they shape how we view the world and what is happening around us. Many SDOH evaluators and evaluations fall under transformative evaluation paradigms because they are based on principles of equality and justice. Frameworks also guide SDOH evaluations and they are either conceptual or theoretical (theoretical implies based on theory, such as one of those listed previously). We reviewed several frameworks, and there are more. Use the frameworks presented as a guide as you develop SDOH focused evaluation plans. The final step in the SDOH plan is **Step 4**, create an evaluation plan and implement it. We presented the initiative planning model as one example of how to outline goals, objectives, action steps, and priorities. Before you complete the model, you will need to know what the literature reports about SDOH and evidence-based determinants. Key questions that this planning process answers include: What are the evidence-based determinants? What are other determinants identified by the community? What will you and the program do to address these determinants? How long will this take? How much will this program cost? What resources are needed? How will you know if you have accomplished your goals in addressing the social determinants? Implementing the SDOH evaluation plan will depend on several factors, some of which have been discussed in this text. RWJF provides an excellent overview on how to implement an evaluation plan (see Chapter 3).

SDOH challenges

By now you know about challenges you might experience while conducting a SDOH focused evaluation. These were mentioned in Chapter 4 but are worth summarizing again because you will likely experience them as you implement a SDOH focused evaluation. First, there is a lack of awareness about the SDOH. This is perhaps one of the greatest challenges that we face as evaluators of public health programs with a SDOH focus. SDOH are not as obvious as poor health outcomes like infectious disease or chronic disease but are underlying conditions that contribute to these outcomes. We do not know the conditions in which people live, their sources of power and strength, but we can see poor health outcomes that come from these conditions. Evaluators play a critical role in shifting towards a SDOH focused paradigm by educating communities and organizations about the SDOH and potential programs that address structural inequalities in the planning process of evaluation.

Another persistent challenge faced by social scientists, evaluators, researchers, and public health advocates is the difficulty of linking SDOH and structural inequalities to poorer health outcomes. To my knowledge, there are four known studies that have addressed SDOH and linked the causal pathways of exposure to a condition and poorer health outcomes. The first study we explored earlier in this text. We reviewed the history of tobacco use, exposure, and advertising in the US, and how policy change was driven by empirical evidence that demonstrated a clear causal pathway of exposure and lung cancer. Evidence required state and federal regulators to monitor tobacco production and sales, and to produce warning labels—but this process took decades even with empirical evidence.

The second study that has achieved this is the Adverse Childhood Experiences Study (ACE) published in 1998. This study was supported by CDC-Kaiser Permanente and is considered one of the largest investigations of childhood abuse and neglect and household challenges and later-life health and well-being (CDC, 2019a). ACEs are potentially traumatic events that occur in childhood (0–17 years). Exposure to violence, abuse, or neglect in the home are examples of ACEs. Other types of ACEs include having a family member attempt or die by suicide, or environments that undermine a child's sense of safety, stability, and bonding. The original ACE Study collected data from 17,000 members of a Southern California health organization. Members completed confidential surveys regarding their childhood experiences and current health status and behaviors. Results from the ACE study have been replicated in multiple communities and contexts of the last 20 years. SDOH evaluations have the potential to transform increased vulnerability to poor health outcomes by addressing conditions that place children and families at risk for ACEs. The CDC recommends these six areas for intervention and prevention of ACEs: strengthen economic support for families, promote social norms that protect against violence and adversity, ensure a strong start for children, teach skills, connect youth to caring adults and activities, and intervene to reduce long-term impacts from exposure to ACE (CDC, 2019a). CDC recommends continued monitoring and evaluation to prevent ACE and improve health outcomes. Earlier in this text we reviewed HRSA home visiting programs for early intervention, screening, and resource referral; these and other programs are upstream approaches that may prevent ACE.

A third study that demonstrated causal pathways between SDOH conditions and poorer health outcomes is the Moving to Opportunity (MTO) housing experiment by Robert J. Sampson (2008). This study selected families below the poverty line and living in concentrated poverty (40% or greater) in five cities during the mid-1990s. These families were eligible to apply for housing vouchers. Families that did not apply were randomly assigned to one of three groups: experimental, Section 8, and controls. This study used an experimental design whereby groups received housing assistance, counseling, and relocation support but the control group received no treatment or support. Results from the MTO evaluation demonstrate five main results that have direct implications for SDOH focused evaluations which seek to improve living conditions and neighborhood effects: adult economic self-sufficiency, mental health, physical health, education, and risky behavior. MTO reported significant positive effects for improved adult mental health, young female education, physical and mental health of female adolescents, and reductions in risky behavior (e.g., crime, delinquency) among young girls (Sampson, 2008). In addition, Sampson reports long-term adverse effects of moving are found for the physical health and delinquency of adolescent males involved in the MTO experiment. One of the main challenges that Sampson and other social science researchers face when conducting SDOH experiences is disentangling the effects of multiple conditions and multiple time points to prove causality. For example, in the case of neighborhood effect, when families moved to improved neighborhood conditions, they also had access to improved education, lower violence and crime conditions, and social norms that support health and well-being. Although some feel that this study does not do enough to answer the "why" questions of causality and neighborhood effects on health equity, it is a start.

Finally, Ludwig and colleagues conducted a randomized experiment to explore how neighborhood environments contribute to obesity and diabetes (Ludwig, Sanbonmatsu, Gennetian, et al., 2011). The Department of Housing and Urban Development (HUD) randomly assigned 4,498 women with children living in public housing in high-poverty urban census tracts to one of three groups. The first group, of 1,788 women, were offered housing vouchers, which were redeemable only if they moved to a low-poverty census tract, and counseling on moving; 1,312 in the second group were assigned to receive unrestricted, traditional vouchers, with no special counseling on moving; and 1,398 were assigned to a control group that was offered neither of these opportunities (Ludwig et al., 2011). A follow-up survey measured data to document health outcomes of height, weight, and level of glycated hemoglobin (HbA1c). Results from this study demonstrate that place matters, and in this case neighborhoods with high levels of poverty, compared to those with lower levels of poverty, were associated with higher prevalence of extreme obesity and diabetes. Results from this study support community-level, place-based interventions that promote health equity.

SDOH solutions

There are many solutions. In Chapter 4 we reviewed the use of a population health approach as a potential solution. We also examined Canada's Population Health Template that outlines how to measure SDOH and interactions between health outcomes and conditions. Briefly, this approach is based on eight key elements: focus on the health of populations, address SDOH and their interactions, base decisions on evidence, increase upstream investments, apply multiple strategies, collaborate across sectors and levels, employ mechanisms for public involvement in strategies and purpose, and demonstrate accountability for health outcomes (Health Canada, 2001).

We also reviewed the CDC's 10 essential public health services. These include the following services that have direct implications for SDOH focused evaluations:

1 Monitor health status to identify and solve community health problems.
2 Diagnose and investigate health problems and health hazards in the community.
3 Inform, educate, and empower people about health issues.
4 Mobilize community partnerships and action to identify and solve health problems.
5 Develop policies and plans that support individual and community health efforts.
6 Enforce laws and regulations that protect health and ensure safety.
7 Link people to needed personal health services and assure the provision of health care when otherwise unavailable.

8   Assure competent public and personal health care workforce.
9   Evaluate effectiveness, accessibility, and quality of personal and population-based health services.
10 Research for new insights and innovative solutions to health problems (CDC, 2019b).

But are these solutions enough? We need programs and research to guide solutions and build health equity.

SDOH programs and research

Previous authors identified solutions for SDOH evaluations and research. These include descriptive studies, longitudinal research, knowledge linked to pathways to interventions, testing of multidimensional interventions, expanding funding that would allow for time to evaluate programs and policies, increasing and growing political will, and a public health workforce that understands SDOH (Braveman, Egerter, & Williams, 2011). Evaluations that employ descriptive studies have the potential to monitor changes overtime and identify social and population factors that impact health outcomes. Results of descriptive studies could move the field of SDOH intervention and program research forward for populations that are most vulnerable and impacted.

Longitudinal research that occurs over a life course is needed, but the investment required for such research will take time and money. Braveman and colleagues (2011) describe the cycles of opportunity or obstacles over the life course, and how these play out in the realms of childhood health, adult health, and family health and well-being. Multiple factors within the living, working, and social–economic environments contribute to opportunities or obstacles encountered. Exploring the impact of social conditions on health over our lives and future generations has the potential to change what we think we know about SDOH pathways, health inequities, and disparities.

Multidimensional pathways also show promise and are needed to direct future SDOH programming, funding, and policy change. Because of the nature of the social environment, and its constantly changing conditions, single dimension studies are not enough.

Research has the potential to increase support for SDOH interventions while informing policy and advocacy efforts that increase health equity. The limited number of studies available (four, listed previously in this chapter) demonstrate that building an evidence base for SDOH is possible but at the same time difficult to achieve. One area that shows promise for linking multilevel exposure pathways is the field of social epidemiology. We briefly discussed social epidemiology earlier in this text, and it is likely that, as the need grows, the utilization of multiple disciplines and expertise will increase.

Although there is work to be done in the areas of SDOH programming and research, the message is clear: evaluators, programs, policy makers, states, and institutions should march forward in their fight for social justice—research is a powerful weapon that can help nations achieve justice and equity for all.

Know differences

SDOH focused evaluations are different from traditional evaluation approaches in public health. Differences are influenced by the history of social inequalities that can no longer be ignored, the underlying causes of SDOH, and the lack of programs and funding that focus on SDOH.

In Chapter 5 we reviewed program examples and scientifically supported evidence from RWJF. A key difference in SDOH evaluations is that they focus on upstream factors that contribute to health. We reviewed the Health in All Policies (HiAP) orientation that is based on building health equity and addressing social, cultural, and environmental determinants that influence health. Several examples of the HiAP were presented, such as the Safe Routes to School National Partnership, the Finnish Initiative, universal access to medical care, American Indian Cancer Foundation, and the CDC's Health Impact in 5 Years.

We also examined programs that are addressing SDOH from multiple intervention points and from the perspective of population health and health equity. A component of several of these programs is that they address racism, discrimination, and implicit bias. These are often silent but strong predictors of health inequality. Programs that are addressing these include the Greensboro Health Disparities Collaborative, Project Implicit, ERASE Racism, and the Dudley Street Neighborhood Initiative.

History of social inequalities in the US

In Chapter 1 we read about the Universal Declaration of Human Rights (www.un. org/en/universal-declaration-human-rights/) that affirms the equal and universal rights to health for all people, irrespective of economic class, gender, race, ethnicity, caste, sexual orientation, disability, age, or location. The right to health has been a topic of interest since the beginning of time, and the history of the US has been plagued by inequality, injustice, and unfair treatment of vulnerable populations. This will not change immediately as the result of SDOH focused evaluations or results. But, when we focus on understanding social inequalities and their underlying causes, then we can move forward toward health equity. From colonization, to slavery, to war, and unfair, unjust treatment of groups because of their racial/ ethnic group or socioeconomic position—we know that health is impacted because not everyone receives equal access to education, housing, healthy environments, support, early childhood development, and health care treatment. We know the reasons for differences in health are deeply rooted in structures and systems that are controlled by those in power. The issue of social inequalities then becomes political in nature, and although this text is not about politics, there is a tremendous need for social service programs that address SDOH and build greater equality in the US and the world. We need new leadership that views every life as equal and important with potential for greatness.

Underlying causes of SDOH

We think we know what the causes of the causes are, but maybe not. Here is an example. We know from previous research that environmental factors contribute to obesity in the US population. Previous research has reported that communities with limited access to healthy foods have higher rates of obesity, and examples were also provided in in this text. Valerie Blue Bird Jernigan and colleagues published results from a multicomponent tribal healthy retail intervention in the *American Journal of Public Health*, the Tribal Health and Resilience in Vulnerable Environments Study (THRIVE) (Blue Bird Jernigan, Salvatore, Williams, et al., 2019). Blue Bird Jernigan and colleagues recruited a cohort of 1,637 Native American shoppers from the Chickasaw and Choctaw Nations. Using a randomized cluster-control study design, the authors explored differences in pre- and post-intervention groups, using individual and store-level outcome measures and standardized survey tools. Individual-level measures included changes in fruit and vegetable consumption, consumption of other foods, changes in perceived food environment, and recall of promotions and subsequent purchasing of healthy foods. Store-level outcomes measured the availability of healthy foods with a focus on healthy fruits and vegetables along with pricing, placement, and quality. This study found that improving access to healthy foods through retail interventions is not enough to change obesity outcomes. Although this was a multilevel intervention, it did not result in the desired impact of reducing obesity and improving healthy food consumption. Interventions must consider the role of policy in changing behaviors, perceptions, and programs as they implement healthy food programs. We must question the causal pathways and exposures that lead to a certain health outcome and ask ourselves the question, "What are we missing here? What should be considered next?"

Lack of programs that focus on SDOH

This text has emphasized the need for additional programs and funding that address SDOH rather than individual or single health outcomes. There is a shift in how programs are being developed and conceptualized and this shift is due to evidence from research and evaluation that demonstrates a lack of health equity in the US and world populations. One of the challenges with writing this text was finding programs and evaluation examples that include a SDOH focus with results. So much of what has been written about the SDOH is theoretical or conceptual, there is simply not enough action, and this is troubling. We reviewed federal and private organizations that are funding SDOH programs—this is encouraging because it shows that SDOH are on the radar of public health and social service agencies. It also means that more programs will be funded that address SDOH, and evaluations will result from these efforts that will build the evidence base for what works and why. We know that a fraction of health program budgets is spent on SDOH initiatives, and most funding is directed toward complex medical care and interventions to treat chronic disease and illness in our world. Additional programs and funding must address upstream conditions and prevention strategies—in doing this millions of dollars and lives will be saved.

Know how to move forward

So much of what we know about health is intuitive. It does not take a HIA, a randomized control trial, or even an evaluation to know what is making people sick in our world. A recent study by Andrew Jebb and colleagues at Purdue University published in the journal *Nature Human Behavior* reports that the ideal individual income in the US is around $95,000 for life satisfaction and $60,000 to $75,000 for emotional well-being (Jebb, Tay, Diener, et al., 2018). This study and many others consistently demonstrate that money is not what makes people happy, well, or satisfied with their lives. On the flip side, we know that a certain amount of money is required to maintain a basic standard of living. This example is important because most of the SDOH literature focuses on moving people from socioeconomic conditions that create poverty into conditions of employment and access to resources. We must be careful if we think that money is the only thing standing in the way of health equity. And, even if people reach the ideal income as reported by Jebb and colleagues, will this make them happy and healthy? Probably not.

The future of SDOH and evaluation hinges on our ability to see things for what they are, and what they are not. SDOH and structural inequalities are deeply rooted in systems and structures that create unfair conditions and disadvantage. This unfairness and disadvantage plays out in generation after generation. When will this cycle end?

Promising strategies

Researchers are working toward a global evidence base for SDOH focused evaluations. This requires political commitment and policies that support health. Increasing knowledge pathways is a first step in building global evidence. In the healthcare realm, strategies that increase access to quality, comprehensive and confidential services, collaborations, and addressing holistic needs of individuals and families are needed (Tebb, Pica, Twietmeyer, et al., 2018). Upstream interventions offer a promising strategy for SDOH evaluation. In Chapter 2 we reviewed differences in program and intervention approaches based on the stream location. As you may recall, upstream interventions target systems change and often involve policy approaches that affect large populations through regulation, increased access, or economic incentives. We used the example of the 1964 campaign by the Surgeon General that advised people about the harmful effects of tobacco use. This campaign is related to decreases in smoking that have been observed for the last 50 years. Midstream interventions often occur within organizations or communities. Midstream interventions are designed to change health behaviors by changing environmental conditions that support them. Downstream interventions involve individual-level behavioral approaches—and these are the most common level of intervention in the management or prevention of disease. The WHO Commission on SDOH report from 2008 recommended three strategies for achieving health in one generation, these being: improve daily conditions; tackle the inequitable distribution of power, money, and resources; and measure and understand the problem and assess the impact of action (WHO, 2008). Healthy People 2020 views SDOH based on five domains: economic stability, education, health and health care, neighborhood and built environment, and social and community context (Office of Disease Prevention and Health Promotion, 2019). Healthy People 2020 provides several example strategies and resources for SDOH evaluation. These strategies and more can help you as you build SDOH evaluations.

Summary

This chapter started with a brief narrative about building an evidence base for SDOH and the role of public health and evaluation in that process. We also reviewed evaluation and program approaches that include a SDOH focus. Next, we explored SDOH challenges and solutions and reviewed research that supports a SDOH approach. One of the most impactful studies of our time is the ACE study. This chapter summarized results from this 1998 landmark study and provided recommendations for future work. Next, we reviewed the history of social inequalities in the US as they relate to the SDOH. There is a lack of understanding and evidence about SDOH, and in this chapter we reviewed a healthy retail intervention to learn more about why multilevel interventions are needed to address SDOH. Although this and other SDOH interventions have not resulted in improved health outcomes, they provide insight and evidence about how to create SDOH programs that address potential SDOH pathways that contribute to poor health. Another challenge we reviewed is the lack of funding for SDOH programs, and the need for a population health approach with a SDOH evaluation focus. This is changing but it is a slow change because it requires people, policies, power, and places to move toward a common goal of health equity for all. As we close this text, know that it is possible to conduct SDOH evaluations and have a positive impact on building health equity.

Points to remember

1 Know that SDOH evaluations have the potential to change how programs are designed, implemented, evaluated, and reported.
2 Draw on existing evidence such as the ACE study and MTO study presented in this chapter to develop and implement SDOH focused evaluations.
3 Consider that programs are lacking, but you can play a vital role in filling this void and moving toward health equity.

4   Consider different strategies and recommendations presented throughout this chapter and text as you begin to develop SDOH evaluations in your work and our world. It matters.

Additional reading and resources

Health Equity and Environmental Justice Collaborative
www.astho.org/Accreditation-and-Performance/Documents/HE-Issue-Brief/CO-Planning-Tool/

Preventing Adverse Childhood Experiences: Leveraging the Best Available Evidence
www.cdc.gov/violenceprevention/pdf/preventingACES-508.pdf

Chapter questions

1   List three SDOH challenges described in this chapter.
2   Summarize results of the ACE study, and describe its relationship to SDOH.
3   Describe future work that is needed in the field of evaluation and research outlined in this chapter. In your own words, write what you feel is needed.
4   Describe the history of social inequalities in the US based on information presented in this chapter and others. What do you feel needs to change in order to achieve health equity and justice?

Activities on the web

1   Review the ACE study resources and best available evidence report (www.cdc.gov/violenceprevention/pdf/preventingACES-508.pdf). What recommendations do the authors have for addressing ACE using a SDOH approach? What information in this document might help you as you evaluate SDOH programs that include an ACE component?
2   Type "Income" and "Happiness" in a web search. What is the relationship between income and happiness based on what you found? How does this relate to your own experience, your own happiness and income levels? Do you agree with what you found or disagree? Why?
3   Review WHO's definition and strategies for SDOH (www.who.int/social_determinants/sdh_definition/en/). What are the key concepts listed, how are these global concepts different than US concepts presented in this text?

References

Blue Bird Jernigan, V. B., Salvatore, A. L., Williams, M., Wetherill, M., Taniguchi, T., Jacob, T., ... & Tingle Owens, J. (2019). A healthy retail intervention in Native American convenience stores: The THRIVE community-based participatory research study. *American Journal of Public Health*, *109*(1), 132–139.

Braveman, P., Egerter, S., & Williams, D. R. (2011). The social determinants of health: Coming of age. *Annual Review of Public Health, 32*, 381–398. doi:10.1146/annurev-publhealth-031210-101218.

Centers for Disease Control and Prevention. (2019a). *Preventing adverse childhood experiences: Leveraging the best available evidence*. Atlanta, GA: National Center for Injury Prevention and Control, Centers for Disease Control and Prevention.

Centers for Disease Control and Prevention. (2019b). *The ten essential public health services*. Retrieved from: www.cdc.gov/publichealthgateway/publichealthservices/essentialhealthservices.html.

Health Canada (2001). *The Population Health Template*. Retrieved from: www.phac-aspc.gc.ca/ph-sp/pdf/discussion-eng.pdf.

Jebb, A, Tay, L., Diener, E., & Oishi, S. (2018). Happiness, income satiation and turning points around the world. *Nature Human Behavior, 2*(1), 33–38. doi:10.1038/s41562-017-0277-0.

Ludwig, J., Sanbonmatsu, L., Gennetian, L., Adam, E., Duncan, G. J., Katz, L. F., … & McDade, T. W. (2011). Neighbourhoods, obesity, and diabetes: A randomized social experiment. *New England Journal of Medicine, 365*(16), 1509–1519. doi:10.1056/NEJMsa1103216.

Office of Disease Prevention and Health Promotion. (2019). Healthy People 2020 goals and SDOH domains. Retrieved from: www.healthypeople.gov/2020/topics-objectives/topic/social-determinants-health/interventions-resources.

Sampson, R. J. (2008). Moving to opportunity: Neighborhood effects and experiments meet structure. *American Journal of Sociology, 114*(11), 189–231. doi:10.1086/589843.

Tebb, K. P., Pica, G., Twietmeyer, L., Diaz, A., & Brindis, C. D. (2018). Innovative approaches to address social determinants of health among adolescents and young adults. *Health Equity, 2*(1), 321–328. doi:10.1089/heq.2018.0011.

World Health Organization. (2008). *Closing the gap in a generation: Health equity through action on the social determinants of health, final report*. Geneva, Switzerland: WHO Commission on Social Determinants of Health.

Appendix A

SDOH evaluation report outline

Front matter

- Title Page: Clear title with date, author, citation, and funding information if appropriate
- Intended use and users: Describe potential use and users of evaluation, when it will be available, and where it can be accessed
- Executive summary: A brief narrative about the evaluation purpose, method, data sources, results, conclusions, and recommendations for future work
- Table of contents: Use headers with page numbers and list figures and tables
- List of acronyms or terms with definitions

Evaluation purpose

Describe the evaluation purpose. Introduce reader to the SDOH, using existing literature and linking that literature to the evaluation focus area. Provide theories and/or conceptual frameworks used to guide the SDOH evaluation plan. Provide a summary of the program. Add details based on the audience that will be reading the report. Consider the following text in the background section:

- Origin and aims of the program
- Participants in the program
- Characteristics of the program and delivery of materials, interventions, out-reach, or other
- Staff involved in the program
- Agency and community role in supporting the program
- SDOH focus and evidence-based determinants

Evaluation method

Summarize the methods used to evaluate the program. At a minimum this section should include the following:

- Evaluation design
- Definition of terms used in the evaluation and references for more information

- Process and/or outcome measures with instruments and data collection procedures
- Types of data collected (qualitative or quantitative or both) and data sources
- Institutional Review Board approvals if necessary

Evaluation summary

Summarize the evaluation findings based on the purpose and outcome. Use text, graphs, charts, tables, and figures to support information presented, but not as stand-alone objects. At a minimum the results section should cover the following:

- Results of the evaluation
- How many people or organizations participated? Were individuals and communities considered vulnerable populations due to their socioeconomic position, geography, social and physical environment, population group, or individually (differential access to healthcare or differential consequences)?
- What were the short-, medium-, and long-term impacts from the program on building health equity among participants or organizations? How was health equity measured? What indicators were used? How were these indicators linked to program activities?
- Did participants, organizations, policies, power, or other conditions change as a result of the program? If yes, what led to these changes?
- Are the differences in results statistically significant? Thematically significant?

Cost and benefits

The cost–benefit section is optional and should only be included if it was part of the evaluation plan. There are several different types of cost–benefit analysis evaluation and the information to include will vary. Generally, cost–benefit analysis evaluations include the following:

- Method used to calculate the costs and benefits
- How costs and outcomes were defined in the evaluation plan
- Costs of the program
- Benefits associated with the program
- Measures of effectiveness
- Unexpected benefits

Conclusion

The conclusion section includes clear and concise recommendations. Write the most important information at the beginning of conclusion. Include the following text in the conclusion:

- Major conclusions of the evaluation

- Recommendations based on results
- Implications for future SDOH efforts, policy and power change, funding, education, health care access, community conditions, and building health equity

References

Select appropriate style and format accordingly.

Resources

As appropriate—these could be used to direct readers to more information about SDOH

Appendices

- Include a copy of the evaluation instrument and other relevant information in the appendix
- Include additional graphs, tables, charts, and supplementary information when appropriate

Notes

Add supplemental information or sources for other materials cited here

Appendix B

Theory of change and logic model examples

The SDOH Example Public Health Education Program Logic Model

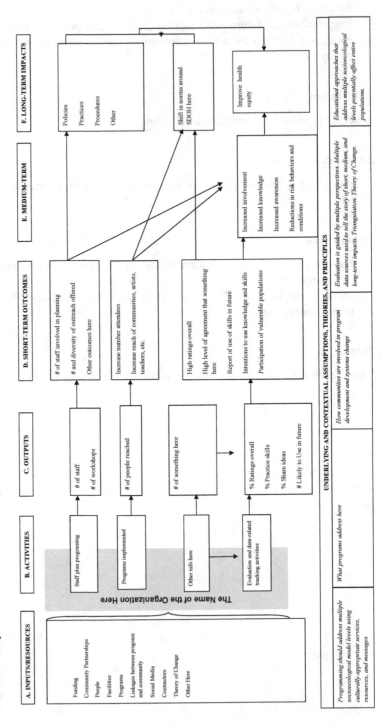

Figure B.1 SDOH example public health education program logic model.

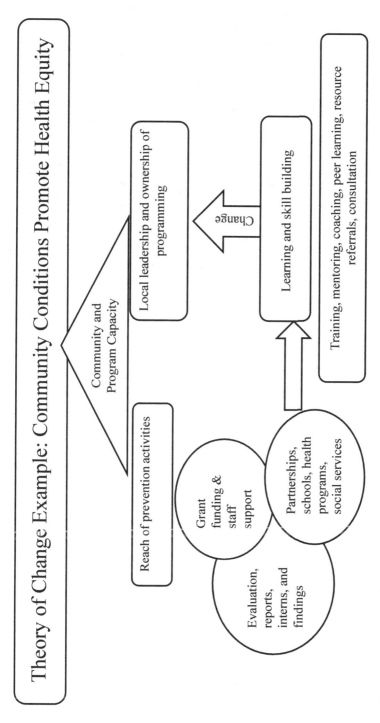

Figure B.2 Theory of change example: community conditions promote health equity.

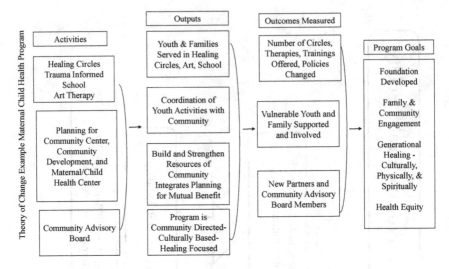

Figure B.3 Theory of change example: maternal child health program.

Appendix C
Health impact assessment guidelines

Health impact assessments (HIA) are a useful tool for determining what SDOH to focus on in a public health program. HIA is a systematic process that uses an array of data sources and analytic methods and considers input from stakeholders to determine the potential effects of a proposed policy, plan, program, or project on the health of a population. SDOH and HIAs are complementary because HIAs help document the distribution of health equity and impacts to health within a population (Quigley, den Broeder, Furu, et al., 2006). Importantly, a HIA provides recommendations on monitoring and managing those effects. Evaluators can play an important role in assisting with the HIA process. There are several types of HIAs in the literature and the type selected will depend on the amount of time that you have, the focus and importance of community engagement, and how HIA data will be combined with other data (from stakeholder interviews to environmental conditions and monitoring data).

Below are the various HIA types and characteristics:

- Rapid HIAs are completed in weeks or months and used for small projects, typically with descriptive or qualitative data.
- Rapid appraisal HIAs require public engagement in the process.
- Intermediate HIAs require more time and money and often involve multi-level and complex analyses and data.
- Comprehensive HIAs may take up to a year to complete, are expensive, and often require new data to be completed (National Research Council, 2011).

If you are conducting a HIA, reporting assessment results should include the following information:

Front matter

- Title page: Clear title with date, author, citation, and funding information if appropriate
- Intended use and users: Describe potential use and users of the HIA, when it will be available and where it can be accessed

- Executive summary: A brief narrative about the HIA's purpose, method, data sources, results, conclusions, and recommendations for future work
- Table of contents: Use headers with page numbers and list figures and tables
- List of acronyms or terms with definitions

HIA purpose

Describe the HIA purpose. Add details based on the audience that will be reading the report. Consider the following text in the background section:

- Baseline health status of the affected population
- Summary of appropriate indicators, including prevalent health problems, health disparities, and social, economic, and environmental factors that affect health
- Discussion of issues that may impact HIA

HIA method

Summarize methods used in the HIA. Here are some potential areas to include in the methods section:

- Describe how HIA analyzed health promoting and adverse health effects
- Describe desired changes in the indicators selected, to the extent possible, in terms of nature, direction, intensity, magnitude, distribution in the population, timing and duration, and likelihood
- Describe how stakeholder input was used to assist with the analysis process
- Summarize data sources and analytic methods and methods used and how stakeholders were engaged in this process
- Outline limitations and uncertainties from the HIA
- Identify limitations and uncertainties clearly

HIA summary

- Summarize the findings based on the purpose and outcome

Conclusion

- Include clear and concise recommendations
- Discuss implications for future HIA and SDOH efforts

References

- Select appropriate style and format accordingly

Resources

- As appropriate—these could be used to direct readers to more information about HIA

Appendices

- Include additional graphs, tables, charts, and supplementary information when appropriate

Notes

Add supplemental information our sources for other materials cited here

References

National Research Council. (2011). Elements of a health impact assessment. In *Improving health in the United States: The role of health impact assessment* (pp. 43–89). Washington, DC: The National Academies Press. Retrieved from: www.ncbi.nlm.nih.gov/books/NBK83540/.

Quigley, R., den Broeder, L., Furu, P., Bond, A., Cave, B., & Bos, R. (2006). *Health impact assessment international best practice principles*. Special publication series no 5. Retrieved from: https://activelivingresearch.org/sites/activelivingresearch.org/files/IAIA_HIABestPractice_0.pdf.

Appendix D

Matrix to document structural inequalities, SDOH pathways, and impact

Structural Inequalities	What is health impact?	Who benefits? Who is negatively affected? Who is not affected/ affected	Pathway of health impact	Magnitude of consequence of impact	Likelihood of impact	Significance (magnitude x likelihood)	Confidence that impact will occur
Structural inequalities, institutional power living conditions, community conditions, risk behaviors and conditions	Positive, negative, not sure, or none	Everyone, vulnerable populations, cumulative impacts	How does health impact occur?	Low Medium High	Possible Probable Definite	Low Medium High	Low Medium High

Source: Adapted from National Research Council (2011).

References

National Research Council. (2011). Elements of a health impact assessment. In *Improving health in the United States: The role of health impact assessment* (pp. 43–89). Washington, DC: The National Academies Press. Retrieved from: www.ncbi.nlm.nih.gov/books/NBK83540/.

Index

Page numbers in **bold** denote tables, those in *italics* denote figures.

Printed in the United States
by Baker & Taylor Publisher Services